JUNG'S SELF PSYCHOLOGY
A Constructivist Perspective

JUNG'S SELF PSYCHOLOGY
A Constructivist Perspective

POLLY YOUNG-EISENDRATH, Ph.D.

JAMES HALL, M.D.

THE GUILFORD PRESS
New York　　*London*

© 1991 The Guilford Press
A Division of Guilford Publications, Inc.
72 Spring Street, New York, NY 10012

Printed in the United States of America

This book is printed on acid-free paper.

Last digit is print number: 9 8 7 6 5 4 3 2 1

Library of Congress Cataloging-in-Publication Data

Young-Eisendrath, Polly, 1947–
    Jung's self psychology: a constructivist perspective / Polly
Young-Eisendrath, James Hall.
        p. cm.
    Includes bibliographical references and index.
    ISBN 0-89862-553-X
    1. Self. 2. Psychology, Pathological.   3. Self pyschology.
I. Hall, James A. (James Albert), 1934–   .   II. Title.
    [DNLM: 1. Jung, C. G. (Carl Gustav), 1875–1961. 2. Ego.
3. Psychoanalytic Theory. 4. Psychoanalytic Therapy. 5. Self
Concept.   WM 460.5.E3 Y78j]
RC455.4.S42Y68   1991
154.2'2—dc20
DNLM/DLC
for Library of Congress   91-6717
                                                         CIP

For my son Colin, who reveals and resists
in just the right measure.
P. Y. E.

For my daughters, Angela and Sherry,
with many thanks for their help
over the years.
J. H.

Foreword

It seems that the best way to comprehend and communicate what is going on across an entire field is to invest oneself fully and passionately, with as clear a head as possible, in a single aspect of it. I say this because Polly Young-Eisendrath and James Hall have produced a work that, responded to fully and passionately, with as clear a head as possible, exemplifies and lays out for the reader all that is most progressive, generous, humane, and effective at the cutting edge of psychology.

The authors make a claim, perhaps the most sustained and systematic to have been produced, for the crucial importance of reading and re-reading Jung in the light of present-day theorizing and clinical experience. Thus, they are partisan. But their very partisanship opens up the way for a reversal of the flow: The assessment of Jung as a constructivist and the assessment of constructivism as Jungian are engaged in a ceaseless articulation. By the end of the book, it is quite impossible to say which viewpoint is the fixed point, the arbiter, the given, the politically powerful—and which viewpoint is the "other" viewpoint, the "second" viewpoint, the one whose place in the intellectual and professional hierarchy is being cultivated and advanced.

Yet the authors *are* making a claim for the importance of reading and re-reading Jung. We should ask ourselves: Why is such a claim necessary? At once, we are reminded of the fact that psychology itself consists of such claims and counter-claims. Psychology is constructed out of them. Psychology exists within a competitive marketplace and displays what must seem to outsiders as incorrigible, incurable competitiveness. Virtually every psychological text, even the most rudimentary teaching aid, is written with an opponent or opponents in mind. The atmosphere within professional psychological societies and departments is charged with a scarcely restrained rivalrous energy.

I feel sure that the omnipresence of competition within psychology has been in the minds of our authors. For, at the same time as showing us that they have a vision of psychology as a potentially unified and coherent field, they chose a comparative and, hence, an inevitably

adversarial model with which to cap their work. I am referring to the
extraordinary achievement represented by Chapters 6–8 of this book
which, for me, truly channel the rivalrous energy for constructive purposes. These chapters contain the case of Jerry, 12 diverse perspectives
on Jerry's material, and a Jungian account in which the authors, to
varying degrees, invest themselves. I feel grateful for, and applaud the
willingness of these authors to let us in on their own disagreements, their
own partially unresolved differences. Something very genuine and full of
integrity is going on here.

Though that section of the book is a *tour de force*, there may be some
who resent what they see as distortion of certain views by the authors for
their own ends. To those who complain of this, I say that I know of no
psychological theorizing, my own included, that does not secretly bank
on such distortion. It is part of the context of psychological theorizing.
Psychological theorizing is contingent upon and constructed out of distortion of the views of the opponent. The hard thing is to argue from one's
guts and yet stay in relation to the opponent. The mixture of tolerance
and tough-mindedness with which the authors work through Jerry and
his numerous "analysts" is a fascinating, pluralistic response to the
difficulties of writing or, rather, making psychology today.

Because of the competitive and argumentative nature of psychology,
Jungians cannot *complain* that Jung's contribution has not received its
deserved recognition. (All's fair . . . etc.) In the light of the authors'
search for a re-reading of Jung, I will focus (all the same) on three
reasons why Jung's contribution to contemporary depth psychology is
often overlooked.

First, the secret "committee" set up by Freud and Jones in 1912 to
defend the cause of "true" psychoanalysis spent a good deal of time and
energy on disparaging Jung. The fall-out from this historical moment has
taken a very long time to evaporate, making the reception of Jung's ideas
in psychoanalytic circles a rough ride.

Second, Jung's anti-Semitic writings and misguided involvements
in the professional politics of psychotherapy in Germany in the 1930s
have, understandably in my view, made it almost impossible for
Holocaust-aware psychologists, both Jewish and non-Jewish, to generate
a positive attitude. There is more to Jung's work than anti-Semitism, but
the evasions in which some portions of the Jungian community often
indulged merely prolonged the problem. Faced squarely, Jung's anti-
Semitism can be assessed both in the context of the time and in relation
to his work as a whole.

Third, Jung's attitudes about women, blacks, so-called "primitive"
cultures, and so forth are now outmoded and unacceptable. He converted prejudice into theory and translated his perception of what was

currently the case into something supposed to be eternally valid. It is the responsibility of post-Jungians to discover these mistakes and contradictions and to correct Jung's faulty or amateur methods. When this is done, one can see that Jung's capacity to intuit the themes and areas with which late 20th-century psychology would be concerned was almost incredible: gender, race, nationalism, cultural analysis, the perseverance and reappearance of religious mentality in an apparently irreligious epoch, the unending search for meaning—all of these have turned out to be the problematics with which psychology has had to concern itself. Recognizing the soundness of Jung's intuitive vision facilitates a more interested but no less critical return to his texts.

In this book, the authors wrestle with Jung's claim for universality and essence on the one hand, and, on the other, his project of the creation of a psychology of cultural difference. They provide a reading of archetype and complex that explicitly joins together the universal and the cultural with an acknowledgment of the tension between. If we want to track the differing psychological experiences and behaviors of different kinds of people, then we must have in mind twin notions of similarity and dissimilarity. For there will be *some* similarities and *some* dissimilarities between the psychological experiences and behaviors of women and men, African-Americans and WASPs, gays and straights, Jews and Germans. It is seductive to account for difference as dichotomy: Women are well-related, but men are emotionally distant. Then we see total similarity or total dissimilarity. In their exploration of what they term "affective-imaginal life," the authors show strength and maturity in standing up for what William James called "the legitimacy of the notion of *some*." In so doing, they give us the bones, and a good deal of the flesh, for a move beyond psychological types or stereotypes of woman, African-American, gay, Jew. Instead, they invite a psychological exploration of the experience of being woman, African-American, gay, Jew at a certain moment in historical time.

Moreover, it becomes clear that such explorations *can* go on in the clinical situation, revealed as the place where personal and political dimensions of psychological experience intertwine.

I conclude with a brief comment stimulated by the sections in this book on the Russian psychologists Luria and Vygotsky, whose work is compared to Jung's. Recently, I had the opportunity to lecture on Jungian psychology in Leningrad and Moscow. I found that, in spite of decades in which Jung's works could not be published legally, many psychologists and non-psychologists were studying his works in secret. What they respected in Jung was his concern for the interplay of individual and cultural factors in psychological functioning and his exposé of the interpenetration of *psychology*, in the form of collective imagery and an apparently *social* situation. These brave Russian readers of Jung appreciated the conception of psychic reality, the argument that there is no unmediated experience, no experience that is not psychologically constructed. For the Russians, Jung's archetypes represented a non-oppressive, anti-totalitarian celebration of the myriad ways in which humanity is joined together by the very differences we display. I hope that they will get a chance to read this book.

ANDREW SAMUELS
Society of Analytical Psychology, London

Preface

Throughout his long career, Carl Jung was passionately interested in understanding the unity of personality. He called this unity the self. Jung conceived of personality more as a loosely organized association of sub-personalities or complexes than as a wholly united structure. Instead of assuming that consciousness guarantees the unity of multiple voices of subjectivity, Jung assumed that unity was hard won and achieved only in adulthood. It resulted from a kind of dialectical balance between conscious and unconscious aspects. It depended on a process of development. That process, Jung knew, was built from early unconscious beginnings into later conscious reflections and capacities to relate. He set the achievement of unity and individuality well past late adolescence because he believed that sub-personalities of early object relations were so coherent and emotionally motivating as to be disruptive of early processes of self-awareness and even consciousness.

Jung was a developmental psychologist without a community of similar thinkers. His discourse is full of "pattern explanation" (Overton, 1990) that uses noncausal or acausal models of metaphor and structure to explain the process or sequence of development. Developmental psychology uses the idea of a continuum or sequence of patterns (e.g., progressive reintegrations) to describe biological, psychological, or social change.

Discourse in developmental psychology often includes terms such as perspective, stage, or frame of reference to represent the momentary organizations of phenomena. Descriptions of these organizations are paired with studies of larger patterns that depict a progressive or directional organization of forms. Jung's idea of "individuation," depending as it does on the differentiation and integration of psychological complexes, is such a model of directional organization. Jung speaks about "self" both as a momentary organization of individual subjectivity (organized as a complex of image, affect, and thought) and as a progressive organizational development.

Jung was ahead of his time in developmental psychology, but more significantly for us, Jung was a "constructivist" well ahead of the advent of constructivism. Constructivism is an account of things that makes special reference to interpretation or belief as a primary aspect of what is taken to be an "object" of awareness. Constructivism contends that what is "factual" is not fixed by something acultural or ahistorical—outside of the perceiver—but is generally influenced by the interpretation of the perceiver. All experience is constructed in a context that includes culture, language, and other persons. We will talk more about this later. For now, we just want to introduce the idea that Carl Jung was a radical constructivist. He believed that the phenomenal world is grounded in emotionally laden images and their interpretive consequences. Constructivism is the context in which we will present Jung's ideas.

It is our purpose to show how Jung's self psychology evolved and can be integrated into contemporary theories of self and subjectivity. We present conceptual idioms and models from Jung's self psychology in the first five chapters. We want to clarify and advocate the clinical use of the Jungian theory of self, as well as show its parallels with other contemporary models of self. We believe that Jung's approach to the topic is unique in the way that it centralizes adult development and self-reflexive processes. In our treatment of a fragment of an analytical case in Chapters 6, 7, and 8, we intend to show two things primarily: that the perspective of self (individual subjectivity) is an essential one for a clinical understanding of adult development (both continuity and discontinuity), and that Jung's model is probably the most comprehensive and adequate model available in this regard.

Rogers and Kegan (1989), in a recent paper on mental growth and mental health, disagree with the central "genetic" hypothesis psychoanalysts hold about mental health: that early stages of development are the most flexible and the most vulnerable and therefore are the most significant for the entire lifetime of development. According to this principle, the most distressing pathological syndromes have their roots in the earliest period of development. Rogers and Kegan believe that this model distorts psychological development, arising as it does from biology. They believe that disruption of later psychological functioning, especially self-reflexive processes, may be as significant for adult psychopathology as is early development. They recommend conceptualizing personality structure more in terms of "the underlying motive of the self to organize experience into a coherent whole . . ." (p. 13). This is what Jung's psychology emphasizes throughout.

Rather than offer a catalogue of Jung's references to self, we have chosen to discuss certain topics that emerge in his most fully realized works on the subject. (Whenever possible, we refer to *The Collected*

Works [CW] for citations of Jung's work.) From the early period of his self psychology (roughly 1916–1944), we draw especially from *Two Essays on Analytical Psychology* (CW 7), in which he first introduced fully the idea of self, although he had used the term earlier in his work on psychological types (CW 6). From the later period (1944–1961), we have chosen the volume *Aion: Researches in the Phenomenology of the Self* (CW 9, II) and the essays on synchronicity, transcendent function, *Weltanschauung*, and the nature of psychic energy—from various volumes. We hope that our selective and systematic approach will entice readers to investigate Jung more fully for themselves.

SOME OBSTACLES TO ACCEPTING JUNG'S IDEAS

Jung is often criticized for being a "foundationalist" or an "essentialist." His psychology is said to be a pursuit of first premises or self-evident givens. Foundationalism is a version of things in which certain patterns or organizations of experience are thought to arise from events outside of any context whatsoever. They are given or inherent in the "nature" of things or the "nature" of the universe. Jung can be construed as a foundationalist because of his pursuit of first principles, such as archetypes, to explain what appears to be universal in human life. Some aspects of Jung's theory do indeed appear to us to be foundationalist in their intent. Jung's theory of acultural principles of Masculine and Feminine is an example of foundationalism. His theory of archetypes, arising from the context of universal human affective-imaginal life, seems to us, however, to be a constructivist project, as we show in Chapters 1 and 2.

We contend that Jung's overall assumptive framework is strongly constructivist, especially in his later work. Some of his foundationalist reasoning is more a product of the cultural biases of Jung's life and times than of the logic or meaning of his theory. Acultural accounts of self, gender, or race now seem wrong and offensive. We think they can be eliminated in a systematic constructivist reading of Jung. In the final chapter, we make suggestions for the future of Jung's psychology that emphasize a more contextualized and relativistic approach to his theory, especially his self psychology. It is our hope that this book will be a first step toward bringing Jung's self theory into line with contemporary constructivist theory and other theories of subjectivity.

The assumption of Jung's anti-Semitism has certainly limited his audience. To put into perspective this accusation, one must examine historical information. This is outside of our purview. We intend here to look at Jung's ideas solely on the basis of their merits as a system of thought, a system that now belongs to at least two later generations of Jungian analysts and theorists, many of whom are Jewish.

"Analytical psychology," the name given by Jung to the body of work evolving from his theories, has been hampered and limited by a too-close identification with Jung's life. His life is neither an ideal to emulate nor a rational argument to oppose nor a foundation for theory-making, from our perspective. It has been treated as each and all of these by biographers and clinical interpreters in various contexts. An attitude of objective reflection on theory, and differentiation from Jung's life, is our orientation to Jung's self psychology. For those readers who would like to study the issues surrounding the accusations of anti-Semitism, we recommend a review by Sherry (1989) of a conference that was held to discuss this topic.

Yet another obstacle to understanding analytical psychology has been the fact that Jung published almost no case material. He was vehemently opposed to using cases from his own practice. Jung was perhaps the first staunch advocate for the "the frame" of analytical process, writing about the essential nature of the "temenos" or container for analytical work. Instead of case material, he used examples from cultural documents, works of art, his own unconscious material and creative works, and patient art. These clinical data are difficult to interpret within the domain of typical practices of psychotherapy, psychology, or psychiatry. His essays tend also to be burdened with elaborate classical references, sometimes to obscure texts in gnosticism, alchemy, and early Christianity. Formal training in Jung-ian analysis provides students and analysts with an appreciation of Jung's allusions to ancient texts and images that continue to evoke our fantasies about love and conflict at the end of the 20th century. To an outsider, however, these allusions may be frustrating and even provocative because they seem irrelevant to the immediacy of thera-peutic work.

One more word about reading Jung's ideas in a contemporary context: Jung (via his translators) uses forms of the male pronoun (he, his, him) to refer to the generic person (including she, hers, her). Rather than note each time this usage appears in quotations (Jung's and others) throughout the book, we simply note here that such usage is offensive in contemporary psychology.

Identifying obstacles to accepting Jung's ideas, in the context of contemporary self psychology, represents our effort to respond to the typical dismissive criticisms of analytical psychology. We agree with many of the criticisms, but we reject any conclusion that analytical psychology is merely a historical chapter of depth psychology, un-necessary for contemporary practice.

OUR PERSPECTIVE

This book is an invitation to both the Jungian community and the larger professional community of psychotherapists and researchers interested in subjectivity. For the Jungian community, we hope to provide a contemporary context in which to read and systematize Jung's ideas. We believe that locating his work within the discipline of constructivist thinking will illuminate and simplify many of his central ideas, as well as put them into a more relative, contextualized framework. For the larger professional community, we hope to awaken interest and desire to know more about Jung's work, as well as to investigate it clinically and empirically.

As we say later, we are convinced that Jung offers the possibility of a unifying paradigm for many aspects of nonreductive psychology— psychology that cannot be reduced to biological functions or learning. Because Jung did not insist on a metapsychology that burdened his clinical theory, and because he was influenced by modern ethology and biology, his model of the psyche can account for complex interactions between conscious and unconscious processes without reducing them to brain functions or learning theories. Moreover, Jung is first and foremost a pragmatic scientist who will accept anything as valid at the level of experience and then attempt to find its truth or falsity in objective examination and empirical study. As a psychotherapist he was both pragmatic and scientific. He was interested in finding what "worked" and then in understanding why it worked. In his later years, he looked back over his clinical practice and used it as a retrospective laboratory to test the theories he was synthesizing from his studies of biology, ethology, and religion.

Our admiration for Jung's perspicacious insights about subjectivity and its development is the motive behind our efforts here. We believe that contemporary practitioners of any form of psychotherapy, but especially of depth psychotherapy, have much to gain by integrating a Jungian orientation. When childhood and adolescence have passed successfully, a person faces a lifetime of meaning-making and purposive action. The symbolic connection to the self is the essential core of well-being and development over most of the lifespan. Jung's self psychology is the most fully achieved model of the nature and course of this symbolic connection.

Acknowledgments

At the top of our list of people to thank is Willis Overton, whose superb talent in editing saved us from a crisis of circularity and restated arguments. Bill's comments and suggestions on a first draft were substantive, friendly, and, most of all, logical. Thank you, Bill.

Bill Overton and Polly Young-Eisendrath are faculty members in the Seminar on Epistemology, Development, and Psychotherapy at the Institute of Pennsylvania Hospital in Philadelphia. Weekly they meet with other faculty, including Harvey Horowitz, Ellio Frattaroli, Howard Baker, and Maggie Baker, and students, all of whom have contributed significantly to the ideas discussed here. In vigorous and joyful debate and dialogue, questions about constructivism and developmental psychology are investigated and resolved in the context of psychotherapeutic practice and research. The authors are especially grateful to the Seminar for the course of readings it provides, and discussions we engage in together.

We extend our appreciation also to Jeff Faude, who was a careful and thoughtful editor and reference librarian. We enjoyed the critical debate Jeff presented regarding Jung's understanding of transference.

The staff of Pendle Hill Quaker Study Center has been generous and gracious over the years of our working there on books and manuscripts. Once again, our friends there provided solitude and company, quiet hours, and comforting smells of bread baking. Thank you, Pendle Hill.

Our family members have endured yet another book. Although they are beginning to take these activities in stride, they sacrifice all the same, especially in being unable to spend weekends together, and occasionally in being left without meals and/or companions at meals. We thank all of you. Polly especially thanks her husband, Ed Epstein, who has been a critic and reviewer of parts of this book, usually at the last minute and without warning.

Finally we thank our editor, Sharon Panulla, who has become a dear friend over the years. Sharon has shown a combination of enthusiasm and helpful advice that keeps us involved.

Of course, we take responsibility for the material presented here. Our friends and colleagues have helped us organize and rewrite it, but we are the authors, and we stand to be corrected for errors and omissions. We look forward to hearing from our colleagues about whether or not we have achieved our aims in presenting a constructivist reading of Jung's self psychology.

Contents

☆ 1 ☆

Locating Ourselves:
Basic Concepts

In presenting the broader picture of Jung's self psychology within a constructivist framework, we attempt to reach both those familiar with Jung's work and those unacquainted. In these two chapters we give a contemporary interpretation of some basic Jungian concepts. Those already familiar with Jung should find a new angle of meaning here as we strive to define and revise his ideas according to our purposes. Those unfamiliar will, we hope, find relatively easy access through comparing Jung's psychology to other depth psychologies, to other theories of subjectivity, and to some of Piaget's ideas. For both kinds of readers, we hope that our conceptual orientation will provide a fresh and illuminating synthesis.

In this chapter, we first introduce the fundamental concepts of archetype and complex in a comparative discussion of Piaget's constructivist theory. We then look at the meaning of the archetypal self in the context of a new definition, one based on a summary of four invariant principles of individual subjectivity. From this base, we develop further some of the basic concepts of a Jungian theory of subjectivity. The definitions we use in this chapter are the product of Jung's later work. In Chapters 2, 3, 4, and 5, we show how these ideas evolved through the development of Jung's theory. Our purpose now is to set the context for later discussions. We begin with the key concepts of the Jungian opus, archetype, and complex.

ARCHETYPE, COMPLEX, AND PIAGET

Archetype means "primary imprint" and indicates a universal predisposition to construct an image, usually in an emotionally aroused state. The dual organization of emotion and image into universal forms is a specifically Jungian contribution to a theory of human instincts. Archetypes arise in human experience and are universal because certain configurations of emotion are ubiquitous in human life. Jung's addition of "image" to the experience of emotional or situational patterns appears to be unique in contemporary psychology.

We can think of "image" here to mean roughly a schematic representation, what might be considered a "pre-operational thought form" within a Piagetian framework (Piaget, 1926, 1932, 1936). Pre-operational thinking becomes initially organized as coherent images in the period of life roughly from 3 years to 6 or 7 years. Thought is organized into idiosyncratic and emotionally infused images. This is the first stage of symbolic thinking; sign is differentiated from signifier. *Preceding* this pre-operational period, in Piaget's model, is the organization of sensorimotor schemes or patterns of action (e.g., grasping and kicking) that are the forebears of thought per se. Piaget, in contrast to Jung, assumes that *action* is the primary or first-order organization of psyche. This marks an important distinction between these two thinkers.

For Jung, the emotionally infused image is the primary organizer or most fundamentally coherent unit of the human psyche. Whereas Piaget emphasizes the repetitive interactions of the infant's body with the environment, Jung highlights the power of emotion to evoke meaningful constellations or symbolic representations at all stages of development.

The period in which image-thinking predominates is developmentally prior to the mastery of syntax in language. Organized images that are the core features of emotionally aroused states are assumed by Jung and Jungians to be more motivating, more powerful, than any attempt to render them in language. Because they are pre-verbal in their first occurrence, and because they are infused with emotion, archetypal images are powerfully motivating and continue to be organizers of psychological experiences (especially in relationships with others) throughout life. Moreover, their meaning cannot be fully encompassed by language and rational forms of thought.

Piaget's theory is based on research and observations of action patterns in the infant's "attack" on the physical world. Jung based his work on psychological research and clinical observations with adults (often in psychotherapy) of the emotional power of image. Whether image or action is primary as an organizer of the human psyche is a point of speculation.

Our own speculation is something like this: Action-schemes lead to cognitive-schemes, concrete thought, and eventually to inductive–deductive reasoning. Images may lead to emotionally based organizations of thought, metaphoric models that eventually develop into representations of complex emotionally motivating schematic meanings. The primary pre-verbal images of childhood never seem to lose their motivating force. They cannot be captured entirely by the basic propositional models of ordinary language, nor can they be defeated by the will to ignore or forget them.

The primacy of affective-imaginal life is the key to Jung's theory of psychological complexes. According to later (1944–1961) Jungian theory, a psychological complex is the primary subjective unit of personality. Its core or "nucleus" (to use the metaphor of an atom) is an archetype. This core is a motivational system of emotion and image-formation that is associated with habitual thoughts, actions, feelings, and other images. The psychological complex is a loosely coherent collection of experiences that are "collected" around the compelling affective-imaginal core. When interpreting a psychological complex in analysis, we draw both on the universal nature of emotional/archetypal life, and on the affective particulars of an individual's history. At the universal level of analysis is Jung's model of collectively shared images (e.g., Great Mother and Terrible Mother) that arise from the ubiquitous character of human emotion.

We will explore this in more detail later, but for now all that is necessary is to grasp the meaning and relationship of archetype and complex. The assumption of universality—acultural and ahistorical—is connected with the ubiquitous meaning of human emotions and the form and function of the human body (although these take on different interpretations within different cultures).

The subjective experience of an unconscious complex can be compared to a trance state; one is "beside oneself" when it is activated. Unconscious complexes are typically called "autonomous" because of the nature of their habitual expressions of impulses, feelings, and actions around an emotional theme. These emotionally charged complexes accrue personal meanings that may originate in preverbal events, but continue with the development of language. When an environmental factor—for instance, another person's habits of speech—evokes an unconscious complex, certain emotions and images are automatically reexperienced. Usually unconscious complexes are evoked in significant human relationships. Many complexes are formed originally in the earliest dependent relationships of childhood and are later reexperienced in other essential relationships.

A central psychological complex, identified with body–psyche being, is the intersubjective experience of "self." As we discuss this in greater detail later, we simply mention here that self is a coherent expression of certain universal features of individuality that are connected with self-conscious emotions (e.g., pride, shame, guilt, and envy). After this complex has formed, recognized first as an awareness of agency and coherence in a particular body, the "ego complex" (as Jung came to call it) is consciously identified with a life history, a personal narrative and identity. Jung observed that this central complex of consciousness and agency is *compensated* or balanced by unconscious complexes. These unconscious complexes overtake consciousness periodically, and a person experiences a powerfully shifting mood ("I don't know what came over me") or an impulse to say or do something alien or at least unlike him- or herself.

The overall organization of psychological complexes in a healthy personality is one of dynamic interplay or dialectical balance. Compensation automatically functions to rectify one-sidedness in ordinary ongoing experience. Jung's model of compensation is similar to Piaget's model of "equilibration" or the balancing of assimilation and accommodation in the ongoing process of experience. When a person is disturbed (i.e., dramatically unbalanced), compensation appears to be symptomatic, and affective-imaginal states seem to overtake conscious, rational thought altogether. Jung believed that forms of psychopathology were attempts of the personality to make "natural" corrections to conscious awareness. If a person consciously suppresses or unconsciously represses too much that is emotionally charged and meaningful, then the system of compensation will "throw up" the "other side," and there will appear an insistent nonrational configuration of action or meaning. Being well connected or related to one's unconscious complexes means living a symbolic life, as we shall see.

BASIC CONCEPTS OF SUBJECTIVITY: PERSONS AND SELVES

It does not seem at all remarkable that every person embraces a self. Each individual constructs a model that organizes subjective experiences into a sense of individual unity. Apparently universal among all human societies is the tendency for persons to order their lives according to their own theories of self or individuality (see Harré, 1984).

Persons are embodied beings who live by theory. They have no difficulty identifying the category "person" (as distinct from object, organism, or animal) after about the chronological age of 3 years (or earlier). This identification is based most likely on the achievement of familiarity with one's own embodied psyche and perceptions of similarity to others.

Persons expect and attribute certain powers and capacities to themselves and other persons, both as regards their relationships and certain expectable aspects of "person-ality." Self as a construct of individuality is one of these universal attributes of persons. As we said above, Jung believed that the subjective organization of self was motivated by an archetype. Individual selves are universal occurrences for all people.

Neither Jung nor Jungians have defined the archetype of self in a way that makes fully explicit its discrete meaning in Jungian discourse. As we shall see, in Jung's work, self can refer to the notion of inherent subjective individuality, the idea of an abstract center or central ordering principle, and the account of a process developing over time.

We would like to establish our definition for what Jung seems to mean by his later theory of "archetypal self," as primary imprint or organizing form for individuality. From the work of Stern (1985), Harré (1989), Spence (1987b), and others we have derived the following "invariant principles" according to which a self is universally organized and sustained. These principles fill out a definition of archetypal self. These principles are inherent in all embodied selves, aculturally, ahistorically. They are core features of a predisposition for unity; they are probably related to the complexity of a specifically human psyche. In later chapters we will talk about other features of the archetypal self, in terms of its emotional and developmental meaning. For now, the following principles assist us in imparting constructivist meaning to the notion of an archetypal self:

1. *Agency:* the experience of personal causation (DeCharms, 1968), authorship of action, intentionality.
2. *Coherence:* the experience of unity or "core being" (Stern, 1985); the collusion of body/psyche; the location of oneself as a point of view with an immediate knowledge of psychical boundaries and discrete bodily organization.
3. *Continuity:* the experience of "going on being" over time (Winnicott, 1965) that provides the functional connections that eventually result in foresight (Sullivan, 1953) and nonverbal and verbal memory as the bases of self narratives (Schafer, 1978; Spence, 1987b) that permit us to connect to the present with past and future.
4. *Emotional arousal:* the instinctual patterns of arousal, expression, and motivational readiness that are relatively fixed systems of subjective relating between persons, and with organisms and things, throughout the lifespan.

These principles of individual subjectivity can be understood as the archetypal self in that they provide the conditions in which a person is predisposed to create an emotionally infused image of subjective individuality. They arise out of personal being, the particular occurrence of a mind–body actor who develops through relationships with other persons. The specific psychological complex organized around the archetype of self is, of course, the product of the family, society, and culture of any individual person. Consequently the nature of any person's actual self may be more or less individual, more or less separate, more or less independent, based on the culture of persons with whom the self is constructed.

Let us look briefly now at some central concepts of Jungian personality theory that involve individual subjectivity. The concepts of *persona, shadow,* and *transcendent function* can all be defined as maintaining coherence, the experience of core being or subjective unity. Coherence is first organized through perceptual and kinesthetic aspects of embodiment, and later as an aspect of *intersubjectivity* with other persons. Emotional attunement and relational empathy are intersubjective components of coherence, as Kohut (1977), Stern (1985), and MacMurray (1961) assert.

The *persona* or "mask" is the Jungian term for the defensive structure or strategy of the ego complex. The persona protects the coherence of individual being through projection, denial, or identification with a role (e.g., as daughter, student, parent, teacher). The persona is a defense especially against threats from others that loosen coherence, or disrupt continuity, caused by lowered self-esteem or other threats (emotional or physical).

Conversely, the *shadow complex* is the "opposite" of the ego—a complex of "not-I" material that is dissociated from acceptable self-representations, and used as a repository of alien (and often unlikable) aspects of the self. The shadow functions also as a defense. A person uses the shadow to defend coherence by projecting or transferring alien-but-familiar qualities "away from the self" to others, outsiders, or the world (e.g., the transference of alien qualities to aspects of the natural environment).

The concept of *transcendent function* refers to a "liminal" activity in which a person makes an identity shift from a typical self-image of the ego complex to a less familiar one of another complex (e.g., to the child complex). This is a process of psychological accommodation that takes place when a person can no longer assimilate immediate experience through the structures of persona and shadow. The transcendent function may serve a temporary function of compensating consciousness or a more developed function of changing a conscious attitude.

The transcendent function is a term to name a psychological reaction to disintegration or lack of coherence. We are disturbed when the integrity of our being seems jarred by our desires or weakened by fears or threats. When the integrity of the personality is threatened, the transcendent function is activated. Often we experience the transcendent function in dreaming when we are induced into doing and being things that complement or complete our waking one-sidedness. Ordinarily, the persona and shadow maintain a balance of assimilating new experiences to the ego complex and externalizing unwanted or alien aspects of ourselves by projecting them into others or the world. Only when ordinary functions fail to work is the transcendent function activated. Jung assumes that the transcendent function (especially as it is activated in dreams and other imaginal states) is evidence of a central organization within the personality that maintains compensation or balance of functions.

Other Jungian concepts of subjectivity can be defined in terms of continuity. Jung's concept of the *ego complex* can be best described as the predisposition to construct a continuous "I" or experience of personal history. Although Jung assumes that intentionality is an aspect of "I-ness," he does not usually emphasize the experience of agency in his ego theory, except in striving for reflective consciousness, the "work against nature." Agency enters into Jung's concept of ego more in regard to the striving to maintain a unified self, than it does in regard to intentional actions or mastery. The motivation to construct oneself as continuous over time, as the "same person" from birth to death, develops as the ego complex with its core of the archetypal self.

Jung describes a tension between the ego complex and the archetypal self. This is a tension between the surface structure of personal identity and the universal development of the individual. Jungians have later called this tension the "ego–self axis." The experience and narration of oneself as a particular and specific individual are in a particular relationship to (may be in conflict with) the archetypal self at any developmental moment. For example, a person may retain "heroic" stories about personal style and characteristics from the risk-taking days of adolescence long after these stories have any place in the coherent body–mind of later adulthood. Jung describes the ego as a psychological complex of ideals, images, feelings, and habits that arises from the archetypal self and that is defended by the persona and shadow, both intrapsychically and interpersonally.

The personality concepts of *anima* and *animus*—as complexes of male femininity and female masculinity, respectively—can also be defined in terms of continuity. Over time, the meaning of gender identity is constructed and sustained by self and others as part of the ego complex. Gender identity is initially reliably recognized and labeled during the period from about 18 months until about 36 months. As Money (1976), among others, has established, gender identity is difficult to change after 36 months. In this same period, the child is establishing what Mahler et al. (1975) call "object constancy" as the basis of an ability to sustain images of oneself and others as continuous and ambivalent. "Gender constancy," the recognition that gender identity will not change, is not fully achieved, however, until the age of 6 or 7 (Ruble, 1983). Gender constancy makes a permanent contribution to the ego complex. One is permanently marked as a member of one of two genders, always to be excluded from the Other. (Other, capitalized, refers to alien or excluded aspects of subjectivity.)

From a Jungian perspective, the repressed identity with the Other constitutes a psychological complex of the one unlike oneself, the "contra sexual" Other. Gender is the symbolic meaning, assigned by culture and sustained through ongoing conversations and conventions, to the two sexes. Repressed gender identity—the partly conscious emotionally charged attitudes, images, and meaning of the Other—is the psychological basis of anima and animus complexes. To maintain that the Other is not-I while constructing the Other from one's own experiences is the paradoxical nature of the contrasexual complex. (Our definition here of anima/animus is our constructivist account of Jungian gender psychology, consistent with the intent of Jung's later self psychology [post-1944] but not with most of Jung's own theorizing about anima/animus, usually considered by him to be archetypes, not complexes.)

In Jungian psychology, envy of the gendered Other is connected with these contrasexual complexes rather than primarily with body parts such as penis or breast. Although differences in bodily structures and functions certainly contribute to the formation and ongoing meanings of contrasexual complexes, they neither wholly explain the complexes nor can be interpreted free of the context of family and cultural meaning.

SOME OF JUNG'S BIASES

Jung's original speculations about self derive from three sources: (1) his clinical work of analyzing adults; (2) his comparative investigations of mythology; and (3) observations about his own subjective experiences, both in his self-analysis and in symbolic life (dreams, fantasies, play, etc.). Even in the early period of Jung's psychology, before his separation from the Viennese Freudian psychoanalytic circle in 1913, he was wary of deterministic formulations and reductions about unconscious processes. Instead he sought conceptual idioms that might "live and work."

For example, in a letter Jung wrote in 1915, he said,

> The core of the individual is a mystery of life, which is snuffed out when it is "grasped." That is why symbols want to be mysterious;

they are not so merely because what is at the bottom of them cannot be clearly apprehended. . . . True understanding seems to be one which does not understand, yet lives and works. (Jung, 1973b, pp. 30–31)

Jung searched for pattern explanations for unconscious processes; he was reluctant to assign any reductive interpretations to unconscious motivations. His wariness about deterministic formulas has both positive and negative effects on his theory. On the positive side, Jung's theoretical models are usually self-consciously hypothetical and constructivist. On the negative side, Jung's models are sometimes internally contradictory and loosely or vaguely defined. In Chapter 2, for example, we will explore some significant contradictions in his formulations of self as the core of an experiential ego complex, and as a universal developmental principle of personality organization over time. His preference for maintaining an attitude of mystery and discovery, especially regarding the spontaneous products of the unconscious (such as dreams), kept him especially tied to adult development. From Jung's viewpoint, only in adulthood are people complex enough to express the unity of personality in a fully creative life.

Throughout Jung's career, he emphasized adult development, and deemphasized "nursery psychology" that seemed to him to be the province of Freud and his followers. During his alliance with Freudian psychoanalysis, Jung held some interest in infant and child psychology, but he replaced this with his investigations of comparative mythology even by the time he parted from Freud in 1913. Notwithstanding his emphasis on adult functioning, Jung's self psychology is congruent with much of the work of later object relations theorists (especially Klein, Winnicott, Fairbairn, Sullivan, and Bion). The object relations theorists derive most of their explanations from analyses of the mother–infant dyad, gathering evidence from observations of this dyad and from adult reenactments of early scenes and meanings, especially in analytic transference. Jung also draws on transferential phenomena (having the character of "primitive" fantasies or desires) in his characterizations of psychological complexes in adult personality functioning.

Jung was drawn neither to observational studies of early life nor to hypotheses about the "clinical child" (see Stern, 1985, pp. 13–15). Explanations that reason "backwards" from clinical experiences with adults to *causal* conjectures about early life were unattractive to Jung. He said, for example, "It may not be superfluous to point out that lay prejudice is always inclined to identify the child motif with the concrete experience 'child,' as though the real child were the cause and precondition of the existence of the child motif" (CW 9, I, p. 161 fn.). We might say that Jung was more interested in the child motif—that is, symbolic and metaphorical images of the child—than the concrete experience "child." Jung used the symbolic child motif often in his interpretations of childhood complexes functioning in adult life. He assumed that therapeutic intervention worked on the current conscious attitude, not on uncovering "the" past or some past. "Neurosis or any other mental conflict depends much more on the personal attitude of the patient than on his infantile history" and "The task of psychotherapy is to correct the conscious attitude" (Jung, CW 16, p. 31). In Jungian therapy, then, the image of a child, in dream or fantasy, often is linked to contemporary events in which the child motif is active. This motif may point to such diverse meanings as new developments, naiveté, freshness or impulsiveness, stupidity, concreteness.

This chapter has provided a basic acquaintance with core concepts of subjectivity in Jung's self psychology. In the next chapter we continue to locate ourselves more completely by presenting Jung from the context of constructivism.

☆2☆

Jung and Constructivism

To introduce Jung as a constructivist we need both background and foreground for understanding the premises of his self theory. Background here is the context of constructivism and how it fits with assumptions of analytical psychology. Foreground is the Jungian model of individuation and the self. Our overall aim in this chapter is to provide clarification about the assumptions of Jung's self psychology, locating it within contemporary theories of subjectivity and development. To this end, we first discuss constructivism and some comparisons of Jung, Luria, Vygotsky, and Freud. Then we turn to a brief review of the evolution of Jung's self psychology in the context of his life and finish with a critique of certain aspects of his self theory. Our central criticism of Jungian self theory concerns the tendency of Jung and some Jungians to describe subjective experiences (such as some dream images or aspects of gender difference) as though they were acultural and ahistorical. This tendency arises in a conflation of subjective and abstract or hypothetical levels of analysis in Jungian theory, leading to a misuse of the Self (the capitalized term that refers to the self beyond experience, the empty center, or the organizing form).

In response to this problem, we introduce "embodiment theory," which links universals and experience. For us, embodiment theory permits a new reading of Jung's ideas and clarifies some of the theoretical confusions that lead to the universalizing of contextually relative experiences and beliefs. Embodiment theory allows us to talk about archetypes and the archetypal Self as universal because they arise in the experiences of embodied persons everywhere. Archetypes are no longer beyond experience.

11

CONSTRUCTIVISM, JUNG, AND FREUD

Questions about how we come to perceive a world "out there" or live by theories of personal being (rather than by a predetermined "adaptation" to an environment) are the core of a new epistemological awakening in psychology. As Jerome Bruner says in a foreword written for Donald Spence (1986), ". . . ours is the generation, perhaps more than any other since Descartes', that has been preoccupied not simply with *nature* or *mind* but with how we know about them, in what sense we can ever have access to their 'reality,' and what the limits of our knowledge are" (p. ix).

These are concerns that preoccupied Jung as well. In light of a progressive shift away from realism and toward "constructivism" in psychology, we introduce Jung's work on self as a constructivist project: a dialectic of differentiation and integration. As Jung himself might have said, "Psyche is the ground of all experience." The structure and image-making activities of psyche provide our only access to the worlds of self and other. Jung was often vigilant in his opposition to *realism* in his theory of analytical psychology.

In its most extreme form, realism is the assumption that the world "out there" is singular, stable, and systematically received or revealed through the senses. Realism has traditionally drawn clear distinctions between perception and illusion, internal and external, and reality and fantasy. From a realist perspective, the brain is a reactive organ that registers and stores and generates representations of "the world," some of which are accurate and others that are not. Philosophically, realism accounts for things (e.g., for sensory perceptions or the nature of the human body) that are assumed to exist independently of any belief or context of practice. The neurobiological theory of depression (i.e., that depression is "really" a neurochemical illness) is an example of a realist belief that is currently popular in psychiatry.

Rationalism, by contrast, assumes that a particular form of thought—logical-sequential—is the superior conceptual method for de-termining the "right interpretation" of experience. The rationalist, in contrast to the realist, understands the brain or mind to participate in constructing the objects of perception or thought. Reality does not emerge from the world "out there," nor is it a product of the brain "in here." For the rationalist, the world is the product of an interaction of activity and thought, of the structuring of stimuli via mental forms or categories. Certain forms of thought are privileged, however, and are assumed to lead to better conclusions about the nature of self and world. Reason is preferred over imagination, metaphors, dreams, and personal opinions in the search for meaning and truth.

Jung's analytical psychology is a rationalist project in certain aspects—especially in Jung's philosophical commitment to Kant. By and large, however, Jung attempts to construct a dialectical psychology that uses a Hegelian model of reason and imagination, of sign and symbol, to depict the balanced interplay of psychological functions.

Freud's psychoanalytic theory, in its original form, is both realist and rationalist. Freud tends to draw sharp distinctions between imagination and reality, illusion and perception, unconscious and conscious. Formulated as biological realism, Freud's general psychology of psychoanalysis emphasizes organic functioning, neuronal and biological processes, by assigning them primary ontological status. Freud's method of interpretation, using associational and metaphorical thought, tends toward a strong rationalism—validating the "true" (that is, latent) meaning of wish and impulse by reconstructing their rational context as historical truth. (For example, the latent dream thought is always a rational sentence.) Thus, Freud and many Freudians insist on the indisputable distinction between wish and reality, between illusion and perception.

Of course it can be persuasively argued—as Ricoeur (1970), Schafer (1976, 1978, 1983), Spence (1982, 1987), and others have—that Freud's method of psychoanalysis is essentially hermeneutic and aesthetic. In order to place Freud squarely within the hermeneutic approach, however, one must "reread" him and eliminate cornerstones of realism and rationalism from his general psychology. The hermeneutic reading of Freud has been sharply criticized—for example, by Grünbaum (1984), Eagle (1984), Holt (1984), and Edelson (1984).

Jung, on the other hand, fashions his entire psychology on the proposition that we exist ". . . only in a world of images" and that "what appears to us as immediate reality consists of carefully processed images . . ." (CW 8, p. 384). His self psychology is rooted in his theory of archetypes, as basic organizing principles of affective-imaginal life. Archetypes predispose all people to create and sustain certain emotionally arousing images. Whereas Jung's affective-imaginal psychology has been difficult to reconcile with many of the mechanistic and drive-related assumptions of psychodynamics, it is much easier to understand within the framework of constructivism.

Constructivism presents a significant challenge to both realism and rationalism. Giambattista Vico (1744/1948) has been named the "father of constructivism" by von Glaserfeld (1984), but Immanuel Kant and the Kantian philosopher Hans Vaihinger (1924) can also be considered as forerunners of contemporary constructivism. Fundamentally, constructivism emerges from the assertion that people actively construct and create their personal worlds. Each person creates models or representations of the world via a structural ordering—a regularity of active thinking or thoughtful action. The active structuring of experience results in a frame of reference or point of view from which the person assigns meaning to new experiences. This frame of reference or representation of "reality" both generates and constrains what is meaningful. This working model of reality does not necessarily reproduce or tap into some external "given" reality. It is rather a method or strategy for actively structuring what is perceived to be a continuous world of self and other(s).

Recent constructivist theorists, on whose work we have drawn here, include Gregory Bateson (1972), Humberto Maturana and Francisco Varela (1980), Heinz von Foerster (1984), and Ernst von Glasersfeld (1984). Other contemporary psychological constructivists—such as Loevinger (1976), Watzlawick (1984), Spence (1982, 1987), and Vaillant (1977)—have contributed seminal ideas for psychodynamic applications of constructivist principles.

The constructivist viewpoint is an endorsement of epistemology, the structuring of knowledge, without an explicit ontology. Knowledge or structuring of thought is assumed to emerge from the natural processes of development of human life as an interpersonal or relational affair. These ordering processes, such as biological maturation and sociocultural expectations, provide the formal boundaries or "constraints" for development of subjective individuality. Although these processes can be observed and traced through the *form* or *structure* of peoples' accounts of themselves, they do not appear directly as a part of experience. This idea of structure is analogous (but not identical) to Chomsky's (1957, 1975) thesis of deep structure in linguistic development. Language, for Chomsky, is an abstract system of rules transmitted through culture to organize the innate capacity for orderly symbolic expression. People develop language neither through learning it nor through innate inheritance, but rather through the practicing of their innate capacities (deep structures) within the established order for symbolic expression (surface structures). Similarly, the structures of emotion and personal being are not static entities but are systems of transformation that have both deep structures that can be traced in historical processes and surface structures that depict a personalized reality.

Take, for example, the assumption of universally differentiated emotions. Categories of primary emotion such as joy, curiosity, fear, anger, sadness, and disgust arise from the universal recognition of facial and kinesthetic expressions. These are the "deep structures" through which emotions are communicated via human activity. Actual expressions of emotion occur within the context of affective particulars that are the "surface structures" or events through which the emotion takes on personal meaning. From this point of view, any particular emotional expression has both a universal and a personal component.

Jung's commitment to the study of cross-cultural patterns of symbolic expression (in mythology, art, and literature, as well as family life) permitted him to study personality in a way congruent with constructivism and contemporary developmental psychology. We construct our worlds through pattern matching, fitting new aspects of our experience into our expectations. Jung studied cross-cultural patterns of symbolic expression (especially connected with the major life transitions, such as adolescent initiation and anticipations of death) over a human lifetime, from dreams, art, ritual, literature, and religion. Jung developed a broad appreciation for the shared meaning systems that contribute to the individual psyche.

Many psychodynamic theories (including even object relations theories) suffer from two problematic fallacies: individualism as a developmental goal and mental separatism as a theoretical context (see Bellah et al., 1985, for further analysis). Individualism, in the sense of independence or autonomy, seems to us to be a distortion of subjective experience in that all personal worlds arise within relationships, especially the worlds of family and work. Models of "the individual" or even of "two individuals" mislead us to think that a single person could be an appropriate unit for understanding human development. Mental separatism is the tendency to believe in individual minds that are housed in separate bodies or brains. Mental separatism has created questions and answers that tend to focus on "intrapsychic" concerns that take place within "one mind." Constructivism reveals the impossibility of mental separatism and recognizes the shared nature of mental processes that arise within an interpersonal field. Jung's later theory of archetypes and self is a constructivist model of subjectivity that accounts for the collective or shared organization of affective-imaginal life.

JUNG, LURIA, FREUD, VYGOTSKY

Jung should be considered, it seems to us, as a forerunner of contemporary structural psychologists or constructivists. He was primarily interested in complex psychological functions and their development through symbolic processes of culture and mind. He was opposed to all forms of reductionism, especially reflex-arc psychology and biological realism. We have found it an illuminating exercise to compare Jung's work to the discoveries of two other early constructivists, the Russian psychologists Luria and Vygotsky. Luria himself wrote that he was "deeply impressed by Jung's *Studies of Diagnostic Associations*, which suggested entirely new ways of applying objective methods to the study of psychological processes" (Luria, 1979, p. 25).

Luria's spectacular career in the study of representational processes was a lifetime search to differentiate the universal from the contextual. His studies in social psychology, his discoveries about cognitive development, and his clinical investigations of brain injuries are all examples of a desire to extend the domain of empirical study to include both the variants and invariants of self. Unabashed in his refutation of reflex-arc and limited behavioral theories of personality, Luria wanted to demonstrate the complexities of human development as it is affected by culture.

Luria and Jung had some significant similarities. For example, they both moved the study of subjectivity from the domain of introspection into the public arena. Luria conducted his studies of complex psychological functions in hospitals, schools, among Russian peasantry, and in other active arenas of the social world. Jung began his psychiatric career and studies in a public hospital where he did active psychological research and psychotherapy with psychotic patients. Later he pursued comparative investigations of ancient societies through field studies and contextual analyses of original texts. Both men refused to erect any psychology of autonomous individualism. Both men refused to study the individual mind as an isolate.

Early in his career Luria observed, "The processes of abstraction and generalization are not invariant at all stages of socioeconomic and cultural development. Rather, such processes are themselves products of cultural environment" (1979, p. 74). Compare this to Jung's statement in a letter written in 1929:

> The symbol never arises in the unconscious . . . but . . . in self-formation. It comes from the unconscious raw material and is formed and expressed consciously. The symbol needs man for its development. But it grows beyond him, therefore it is called 'God,' since it expresses a psychic situation or factor stronger than the ego. (Jung, 1973b, p. 62)

Although their styles of expression are quite different, both Luria and Jung were committed to a cultural and symbolic context to account for the complexity of higher psychological functions. The interplay of the individual and the universal, the variant and the invariant, was the stage on which both theorists set their work.

Luria insisted, and Jung would agree, that "the basic units of psychological analysis were functions, each of which represented systems of elementary acts that controlled organism–environment relations" (1979, p. 9). Moreover, Luria averred that emotion would be the keystone to understanding continuity and discontinuity in consciousness.

In his work on lie detecting in criminals, Luria discovered that both normal and criminal subjects

> influenced by strong emotions adapted to each new situation in a unique way and did not settle into a stable reaction pattern. Not only did the subjects have unstable motor and speech responses when considered separately, but they seemed unable to create a single functional system that included both motor and speech components, often delaying the speech components of their reactions. (1979, p. 35)

Luria's description and investigation of such "emotional complexes" was based directly on Jung's association experiments (Jung, CW 2): studies of affective components of word associations, applied to normal subjects, criminals, and hospitalized mental patients.

Whereas Jung and Luria developed psychologies of subjectivity and consciousness (hand in hand with theories of unconsciousness), Freud avoided speculations about self. Freud's commitment to biological determinism tended to prevent him from asking questions about the nature of subjectivity. Because Freud assumed the fundamental motivational power of biological drives, he was minded to perceive subjective experience as adaptation. Freud could not postulate a synthetic function of self other than the biological integration of perceptions and motor functions. His late work on ego and anxiety (Freud, 1926/1959) introduced the study of consciousness. His theory of "signal anxiety," developed in response to originally real dangers in the environment, and his tripartite model (ego, id, superego) of psychological functions (Freud, 1923/1961) mark the beginning of Freud's interest in the study of consciousness late in his career.

Freud's later ego psychology and its extensive development within psychoanalysis (e.g. Hartmann, 1958; Jacobson, 1964) have provided a model of subjective agency, articulated especially as the concept of "mastery" in ego psychology and the psychology of defensive structures. Models of coherence, continuity, and emotional arousal (not reductive drive theory) have been more difficult to organize within classical psychoanalytic approaches to subjectivity.

Object relations theory has of course corrected this imbalance, and contributed a theoretical understanding of coherence and continuity to the psychoanalytic literature. Contemporary infant and affect research has also contributed a full-blown theory of emotional arousal (core motivational states). Modern psychoanalysis speaks fully to subjective individuality, but Freud did not.

Jung never accepted, nor even seriously entertained, Freud's commitment to biological determinism as sufficient explanation for the characteristics of self experiences. Neither did Luria. Instead, Jung and Luria proposed psychological theories that would account for the "heights" of human development, the function and evolution of the highest forms of cultural expressions depicting an enormous range of creative expression within a collectivity of persons. As Luria says, his studies proceeded from the "belief that human beings' higher psychological functions come about through the intricate interaction of biological factors that are part of our physical makeup as *Homo sapiens* and cultural factors that have evolved over the tens of thousands of years of human history" (1979, p. 56). Jung also opposed any attempt to reduce human culture to biological determinants and/or to imagine human consciousness as an *epiphenomenon* of physical existence.

In Russia in the mid-1920s, Vygotsky, teacher and colleague of Luria, specifically identified his goal for psychological research as the study and description of complex mental and psychological functions. As Luria described Vygotsky's position,

> man is not only a product of his environment, he is also an active agent in creating that environment. The chasm between natural scientific explanations of elementary processes and mentalist descriptions of complex processes could not be bridged until we could discover the way natural processes . . . intertwined with culturally determined processes to produce the psychological functions of adults. (1979, p. 43)

Vygotsky's commitment to the study of more complex functions, and especially the psychological functions of adults, is remarkably similar to Jung's work of the same period.

Jung approached his study of consciousness with the presupposition that self-reflection and adult intentionality emerge from an a priori structure, an intelligence that is unconscious. Quoting from a passage in Vygotsky's *Thought and Language* (published in an English translation in 1962), Bruner (1986) stresses Vygotsky's similar emphasis on the "transformation" of simpler mental functions:

> Consciousness and control appear only at a late stage in development of a function, after it has been used and practiced unconsciously and spontaneously. In order to subject a function to intellectual control, we must first possess it. (quoted in Bruner, 1986, p. 73)

The a priori possession of psychological functions, the nature of unconscious organization, preoccupied Jung from the beginning to the end of his career.

Shortly after Vygotsky's premature death in 1934, the Russian authorities suppressed his work because they found it "too mental, too idealist" (Bruner, 1986, p. 71). Jung's work was also suppressed and purged from psychoanalytic annals because he was considered too esoteric, idealistic, and unscientific. The accusations against Jung arose principally from the debate over the singularity of sexual libido as the motive for human development.

According to Jung (1961, p. 150), Freud insisted on an untenable "dogma" in which sexuality would be the central force and organizing principle for human motivation and creativity. All cognitive development was to be understood as beginning with the desire for release from sexual tension. Jung, even in his first acquaintance with Freud's work, found the "pleasure principle" to be a barrier to understanding human motivations and instincts. Although Freud also later rejected this singular motive, he did not formulate a model that allowed for a full diversity of human instincts.

Contemporary psychoanalytic theorists now tend to embrace a more complex theory of motivation than Freud did. Whether motivation is thought to arise from the conflicts of wishes and desires or from the emotional configurations of early object relations, contemporary psychoanalytic theorists often agree with the theoretical positions taken by Jung in regard to the complexity of human motivations, although they are largely ignorant of Jung's work. The actual similarity between many of Jung's ideas and contemporary psychoanalysis is striking to those familiar with Jung's work. As Roazen (1976) says in *Freud and His Followers,* "Few responsible figures in psychoanalysis would be disturbed today if an analyst were to present views identical to Jung's in 1913" (p. 272).

Jung's insistent commitment to understanding more complex or higher functioning (without reducing it to biology) led to prescience in advancing "modern" principles of psychoanalysis. Jungian analyst Samuels (1985) shows, for instance, that no fewer than 15 major contributions made originally by Jung have been rediscovered by psychoanalytic thinkers who give no credit to Jung. The avoidance of the Jungian corpus on self seems to be an unfortunate and unnecessary blind spot in contemporary depth psychology.

JUNG'S SELF PSYCHOLOGY IN THE CONTEXT OF HIS LIFE

Some obstacles to understanding Jung's self psychology arise from the changes in the theory over Jung's lifetime. In order to clarify the development of the theory, we introduce a brief account of the historical evolution of Jung's self theory in terms of his life and interests.

Jung made a substantial theoretical shift from his early work on self (1914–1944) to his later position (1945–1961). We have taken the year 1944, when Jung was 69 years old, to be a convenient marker for this shift. Coward (1985) traces Jung's early interest in self theory to yoga, particularly Patanjali's *Yoga Sutras*. Stimulated initially by Wilhelm's translation of a taoist text, *The Secret of the Golden Flower*, Jung (CW 13) wrote a foreword to the work and introduced an Eastern point of view on subjectivity. In this introduction, Jung talks about the notion of an ego "circumambulating" the self—being loosely organized by the boundaries of the self. The self is the "empty center" or core of the personality that is particularized through the ego.

In 1938 Jung traveled to India for the 25th anniversary of the University of Calcutta. By this time he was submerged in Western texts. His commitment to the study of alchemy and gnosticism was so strong by then that he did not even disembark his ship when it stopped in Bombay, preferring to stay aboard in order to continue his immersion in Latin alchemical literature (Jung, 1961, p. 284). Alchemy and gnosticism had preempted other inspirations for Jung's metaphors of subjectivity.

The years just preceding 1944 were a time of Jung's maximal involvement in the professional world. In 1938, he gave a presidential address to the 10th International Medical Congress for Psychotherapy at Oxford, England (CW 10), and presented his Terry Lectures (CW 11) at Yale University in the United States. While the storm of World War II was gathering in Europe, Jung was immersed in Latin scriptures: "The Spirit Mercurius" and "Paracelsus as a Spiritual Phenomena" (CW 13) are essays written in this period.

In 1944, Jung accepted a chair in medical psychology at the University of Basel. While preparing to assume this honor, he broke his foot and then suffered a severe heart attack. During the convalescence from this illness, at the height of his intellectual career, Jung made a major shift in his work at the age of 70. For a period of 3 weeks, Jung encountered mysteries and visions described in his autobiography as "the most tremendous things I have ever experienced" (Jung, 1961, pp. 289–298). He attributed great value to these events, so much so that he assumed they were as "objective" as the phenomenal world (see Jung, 1961, pp. 289–298). Much of Jung's later theorizing about the nature of psychological structures, especially about the interface between psyche and world, was motivated by the forceful impressions of these visions.

Jung's illness was followed by an extremely fruitful period of psychological study, lasting until the end of his life in 1961. He himself remarked that his "principal" works were written only after this illness. He became more interested in the collective implications of psychology and in the study of ethology, biology, and comparative religions. Whereas his earlier works focused on the psychology of the individual, the later ones, on the phenomenology of self and synchronicity, for example, were devoted more to collective themes.

EMBODIMENT THEORY AND JUNGIAN EPISTEMOLOGY

As a first step in presenting a constructivist reading of Jung's self psychology, we borrow from a current theory of knowledge called "embodiment theory" (e.g., Johnson, 1987). Embodiment theory helps us avoid both Platonic idealism and Kantian mentalism in interpreting Jung's theory of archetypes, especially the self. Rather than assuming that mental categories and knowledge are either derived from inherent structures of the universe or the mind, Lakoff (1987), Johnson (1987), and others (e.g., Overton, 1990; Csikszentmihalyi & Larson, 1984; Lakoff & Johnson, 1980) take the position that basic categories of mental experience are derived from human interactions with an environment in flux.

The size and nature of the human body impose ubiquitous constraints on the human psyche. Certain apparently universal properties of thought and experience emerge not objectively in the world independently of any being but rather in interaction with human and other environments.

As Lakoff (1987) says in describing a "basic-level" (his term) category of thought:

> Perhaps the best way of thinking about basic-level categories is that they are "human-sized." They depend not on objects themselves, independent of people, but on the way people interact with objects: the way they perceive them, image them, organize information about them, and behave toward them with their bodies. (p. 51)

A basic-level category is a conceptual unit that is evident in all languages and cultures. It is fundamental to human knowledge. The following characteristics distinguish a basic-level category: it provides fast identification (single mental image or easily perceived shape); it is associated with a general level of motoric interaction with the environment; it is communicated in the shortest and most commonly used words; it is first learned by children and is first to enter the lexicon of language formation; and it organizes most of our semantic memory (most attributes of categories are stored at this level). Basic-level categories are more frequently and easily used in human communications, and they are preferred over their "superordinate" or "subordinate" counterparts.

Lakoff (1987, p. 46) gives the following examples of basic-level, super-ordinate, and subordinate categories:

Superordinate	animal	furniture
Basic level	dog	chair
Subordinate	retriever	rocker

Basic-level categories are directly connected with our embodied per-ceptions in the ease with which we can use them to make and retain categories of thought.

Lakoff (1987) demonstrates extensively and persuasively, in a re-view of linguistic and psychological research, that basic-level categories are shaped through the properties of an embodied point of view and point of action on the world. The universal form of the human body is an ever-present frame for our subjective experiences of ourselves, others, and the world. Embodiment provides both affective–motivational sys-tems and schemata for organizing perceptions and actions of a body in space.

Lakoff's (1987) system allows us to consider the archetypal self to be a categorical product of human embodiment, a universal form for organizing an attitude of individual subjectivity. Embodiment theory makes an explicit link between the ubiquitous features of subjectivity and the actual experiences of embodied persons. This approach moves away from assumptions of ideal forms, realms, or categories of the mind that lie "behind" experience, and thus encourages a different way of looking at universals in the human sciences. Embodiment theory is not biological reductionism (nor even related to it) because its categories emerge from analyses of meaning systems and the ways in which people construct meanings from experience.

In using Lakoff's model of basic and other categories for our own purposes, we decided to sort out the terms that relate to individual subjectivity in ordinary conversation. We came up with the following account:

Superordinate	self
Basic level	person
Subordinate	personal identity/individuality

The primary and immediate experiential category of individual sub-jectivity seems, using the logic of embodiment theory, to be "person." The category of "person" as an embodied individual in a certain form and with expectable powers is easy to identify. Persons are never confused with corpses (just bodies) or with minds or spirits; the category is easy to use.

Self, on the other hand, is more abstract and secondary. A self is acquired within a culture of persons. Although the universal or archetypal self—agency, coherence, continuity, and emotional arousal—is associated with each individual self in a particular way, it obviously derives from embodiment and the primary ground of being a person. The archetypal nature of subjectivity is experienced directly by the person called "self," and is inferred in other persons, through observations, report, and experience. The meaning of person (embodied being) does not shift by culture or context, but the meanings of self shift profoundly by culture and context.

SELF AS METAPHOR, SELF AS DESIGN

Lakoff (1987) presents four models or paradigms of thought that are used for sorting experiences into categories: propositional, image-schematic, metaphoric, and metonymic. In order to apply the metaphoric model to our understanding of the archetype of self, we need a brief introduction to Lakoff's system. As he describes them, metaphoric models are mappings of propositional and image-schematic material from one domain of experience onto another in order to explain the new domain.

Propositions are the bases of much of our knowledge structure. They specify the component parts of experience, their properties and the relations among them. Propositions are "proposals" or "hypotheses" that can be tested, believed, doubted, or denied. An example of a propositional model is the idea that all forms of conflict (interpersonal, conversational, and intrapsychic, for example) fit into a model of danger, tension, and opposition. When a propositional model is used as metaphor, a part or whole of the overall proposition—for instance, war is conflict—is used to map a different domain of experience—for instance, debate—and the characteristics of the first are attributed to the second: debate is dangerous, adversarial. We understand "self" as a propositional metaphor for that person in the world to whom we can attribute the archetype of subjectivity by direct experience. Other persons are "not-self" because we perceive them primarily through observation, not direct bodily experience. Yet, we readily infer selves in others because we assume that all kinds of persons fit into the model of individual subjectivity, although only one person (myself) experiences it directly.

Image-schematic metaphors, according to Lakoff (1987), are prototypical visual or spatial representations that derive from interactions

with the physical and cultural environment. Images of containers, inner/
outer, linear shapes, trajectories of movement and the like are examples
of image-schematic models that may relate to the physical geography of
the human body. Image-schematic models, like propositions, are used
as metaphors to map from one dimension of experience to another. A
particular model, the body = container, is often used to map psychological meanings of the self. The container metaphor may be used to suggest
that the self is either "within and internal" or the "container" of parts of
the personality.

My "self" is my point of view and agency for action. These propositions organize and explain a complex range of perceptual and causal
experiences. The conceptual schemes of being an agent and having a
coherent point of view are mapped onto the model of self. Any particular
propositional model for the self is acquired in a culture of persons.
Similarly, the image-schematic model of the body in space, inside and
outside, above and below, etc., is used as a metaphor of self. The self is
generally referenced to "my" body and thought to be "inside" some part
of the body (e.g., head or heart), or is conceived as the center of activity
of the body.

The archetype of self, then, can be considered a universal metaphor
that is used to map invariants of subjectivity back and forth between
embodied experiences of oneself and inferred experiences of other selves
(symbiosis, emotional attunements, observations, linguistic and other
forms of communication). The full use of this metaphor occurs only after
individual subjectivity can be recognized and filled out by the propositional models of the culture in which the person is developing.
Gradually each person comes to use the metaphor of self as others do.

When Jung and Jungians use "the Self" to mean a universal organizational structure, such as the "empty center" or the totality of personality, they are not using a metaphoric model arising from experience. This
second usage is more like what Lakoff (1987) calls a "metonymic
model": a category of thought in which a part stands for a whole (as a
"head" of cattle stands for the whole animal). This metonymic usage is
confusing because it refers both to the abstract design or process (e.g.,
individuation around an "empty center" of personality) for the development of self and to the thing that is developing. The recommendation of
some Jungian scholars to capitalize this metonymic use (the Self of
totality or wholeness) to distinguish it from the metaphoric/experiential
use of self (explained above) does not clarify the epistemological problems that arise from these two different meanings of self.

The conflation of experiential and abstract meanings of self results
in a blurring of levels of analysis in Jungian theory. Jung and Jungians
frequently blur the distinction between "functional" and "design" levels

of analysis in clinical and theoretical discourse. Functional analysis or interpretation involves the meaning of particular events or experiences. This is the typical level of analysis used to understand a psychological complex as it is enacted in therapy, for example. Such meaning is contextualized historically and culturally and is embedded in peoples' actual experiences.

At the level of design (see Dennett, 1987) one is dealing with abstract patterns or structures that cannot be experienced. They can only be deduced by studying forms implicit in experience. At the design level, predictions are made that people or events will behave or emerge in the way they were "designed" to do. Jung's concept of individuation is a design level of analysis. No one can experience the design of personality. Similarly, no one can experience the Self because the term refers to an abstraction, a hypothesis.

Sometimes when Jung discusses contextual features of self (for example, how it is represented in a dream), he fuses functional and design analyses. He writes as though there is no distinction between immediate subjectivity and universal design. Dreaming of a mandala, for instance, *is* dreaming of the Self. This kind of blurring can become a slippery slide from personal and cultural experiences of subjectivity (self/other) to universal pronouncements about the "true nature" of individuality. Assumptions about the given nature of gender difference (such as categories of masculine as Logos and feminine as Eros) or about universal representations of the self (that a circular image always represents the Self in dreams, for instance) are examples of foundationalism that emerge in blurring the subjective and the universal. When the experiential and design levels of analysis are not differentiated, and when the term "self" refers both to experiences of subjectivity (universal or personal) and to inferences about the development of selfhood (that subjectivity unfolds in a particular pattern or organization), then it may seem only natural to speak as though a person could immediately experience her/his own "organizing principle." We will say more about how this kind of error occurs in Jungian theory, and about our suggestions for correcting it in the final chapter.

Constructivism as an orientation to theory demands a certain kind of thinking—centralizing context, belief, and interpretation. The human body and its constraints are parts of all contexts in which persons live. Embodiment theory is an epistemology that fits well with constructivism and provides a clarifying link between universals and particulars in self psychology. We will align Jung's psychology more fully with these contemporary approaches in later chapters, but in the next chapter we set out some of Jung's early interpretive strategies for explaining the interplay of psychological complexes in the process of individuation.

☆ 3 ☆

Individuation as Ordering Principle of the Self

Jung described the process of individuation in adult life as a recognition of "psychic totality": inner psychological conflict and the balance of conscious and unconscious processes. Individuation essentially means the differentiation and reintegration of unconscious psychological complexes so that a person becomes aware of the overall dialectical nature of personality. Jung believed that this awareness, in itself, would permit the decentralizing of the ego complex, a decentering from the "just so" world of childhood.

One of Jung's earliest (1928) definitions of individuation shows its contrast with a philosophy of *individualism.*

> Individualism means deliberately stressing and giving prominence to some supposed peculiarity rather than to collective considerations and obligations. But individuation means precisely the better and more complete fulfillment of the collective qualities of the human being. . . . The idiosyncrasy of an individual is not to be understood as any strangeness in his substance or in his components, but rather as a unique combination or gradual differentiation, of functions and faculties which in themselves are universal. (CW 7, p. 174)

The process of individuation reveals the universal characteristics of human development, especially in adult development. As Jung says, this process "seems to stand in opposition to self-alienation" (CW 7, p. 173). Hence, individuation leads to the dissolving or understanding of grandiose or devaluing childhood fantasies, identified with self or projected onto others. Individuation should ultimately result in greater consciousness of the full range of conscious and unconscious impulses, actions, and symbolic meaning.

In discussing the process of individuation in this chapter, we attempt to locate Jung's theory within contemporary research on lifespan structural development. Our first step is to understand the psychological beginning of individuation in the experience of neurosis or self-division. Although Jung talked about individuation beginning both at birth and in the experience of self-division (the recognition of inner conflict), we have chosen to discuss it here in regard to self-division. Development begins at conception, but the process Jung calls "individuation" seems to be more consistently connected with self-reflexive symbolic transformations than with earlier developmental processes.

THE PURPOSE OF NEUROSIS

The experience of self-reflective consciousness depends specifically on a person's ability to differentiate from parental complexes that are the shapers and movers of one's original sense of identity, one's initial being in the world. In adolescence and adulthood these parental complexes tend to overtake conscious subjectivity with ideas, moods, and habits that are seemingly "autonomous," i.e., not subject to one's will. As long as parental complexes remain the unquestioned structures on which "reality" is situated, either through identifying with them or through projecting them onto others (including the actual parents), a person is unable to become a psychological individual—one capable of self-reflection, personal responsibility, and personal meaning.

Neurosis or personal suffering can open the door to psychological wholeness, as Jung describes it, if a person can develop greater integrity through understanding and taking responsibility for psychological conflict. The psychological symptoms of childhood difficulties or failures of adequate parenting (and all parents more or less fail to be adequate at some stage of a child's development) are frequently expressed as excessive self-pity, envy, and/or self-aggrandizement in adulthood.

Winnicott (1965), Kohut (1971, 1977, 1984), and Kernberg (1976) have described the pathological condition of narcissism as a particular symptom of an inadequate parental environment resulting in the formation of a "false self" or a defensive presentation of self. Although Jung has a theory of pathological narcissism (when defenses are excessive, see below), he also normalizes the "false self" as a feature of development in adolescence and early adulthood in his theory of the persona.

Idealizing reflections of oneself and defensive denial of one's darker motives are the *via regia* of the persona. The persona is a defensive structure that permits people to function as individuals prior to understanding (or being aware of) motives, intentions, responsibility, and other aspects of psychological individuality (CW 7, p. 157).

In personality development, the persona emerges most forcefully in adolescence with the experienced need for a personal identity. The persona, as a defense against interpersonal threats and lowered self-esteem, is structured from parental introjects, social role responsibilities, and peer expectations. In growing up, the child is repeatedly told how she/he looks, feels, and should be. When self-searching adolescents come to the question "Who am I?" (a question that cannot be asked prior to adolescence and the ability to reflect on oneself), they answer in terms of the persona—in terms of demographic features, social roles, and family values that may be imitated or opposed.

Under ordinary conditions, without acute childhood trauma, the persona functions in adolescence and early adulthood to be an "as if" personality. The persona is normally structured as the "best possible face" that can be taken by the developing adolescent. Weaknesses, fears, real or imagined flaws are "hidden" by the persona. The North American adolescent constructs her/his persona as if she/he had a "unique" or "individual" identity. The persona meets the demand to be an individual and have a social and cultural identity *before* these aspects of self have been understood by the developing person.

Jung emphasizes the necessity for Europeans and North Americans to "feign individuality" in adolescence and early adulthood. Feigned individuality is the identification of the self with the persona. During the period of feigned individuality, the experience of individuality is a more or less arbitrary segment of the collective psyche, according to Jung.

> It consists in a sum of psychic facts that are felt to be personal. The attribute "personal" means: pertaining exclusively to this particular person. A consciousness that is purely personal stresses its proprietary and original right to its contents with a certain anxiety, and in this way seeks to create a whole. . . . It is . . . only a mask of the collective psyche, a mask that *feigns individuality*, making others and oneself believe that one is individual. . . . (Jung, CW 7, p. 157, italics in original)

This persona passes for individuality which is neither understood nor experienced.

Accompanying the persona is a *shadow* complex, the psychological opposite of consciously held values. The shadow is structured by emotionally arousing themes that are aspects of the self from which the person consciously or unconsciously dissociates, unconsciously projects, or knowingly deplores. Repression and other defenses (such as projection, passive aggression, or reaction formation) are used to deal with threatening shadow themes within one's self-reflections and relationships. The shadow complex is a fundamentally "not-I" subpersonality. During early life and childhood years, persona/shadow themes are shaped by verbal and nonverbal communications, traumatic events, identifications with siblings and parental figures, as well as by friends and social/role expectations. Aggressive, feared, or simply disclaimed ideas and images of oneself are excluded from conscious identity because of their alien nature.

When the persona is excessively rigid or defensive, the shadow is "split off" from conscious identity, inaccessible to ordinary awareness. The persona then develops into a pathological false self, leaving the shadow entirely out of awareness. A heavily defended persona may be an outgrowth of primary childhood trauma, such as sexual abuse or serious injury. It may result from a failure in primary empathy of parents or from other disabilities in the psychological or physical aspects of growth. It is always accompanied by a powerfully negative shadow that is difficult to confront. The heavily defended persona is a pathological false self, different from the simple conformity of an unanalyzed persona.

In cases of nontraumatic development, the young adult feigns individuality through successful conformity to family and society. In order to progress towards authentic individuality, a person must break the initial identification with the persona and take responsibility for one's own shadowy meanings. (Not all adults take this developmental step.)

This step is the beginning of a dialectical relationship with oneself. If one is able to differentiate oneself from the "social look"—the way one tries to appear—one can become capable of insight into one's own complexes. After the persona has been clearly distinguished from the experience of subjectivity—differentiating both pretense and role from actual felt experiences—then a person has the possibility of seeing through appearances and understanding the functions of collective individuality.

Neurosis is frequently the beginning of authentic individuality. Jung uses the term "neurosis" loosely, as does Freud, to indicate broadly all nonpsychotic psychological disturbances. (By contrast, we would now distinguish between neurosis and personality disorders.) These are manifested in relational or other symptomatic problems that interfere with intentional control. Although neurosis is distressing and impedes wellbeing, it also opens doors to new awareness and to insight about motivation and meaning.

Neurosis is intimately bound up with the problem of our time and really represents an unsuccessful attempt on the part of the individual to solve the general problem in his own person. Neurosis is self-division. In most people the cause of the division is that the conscious mind wants to hang on to its moral ideal, while the unconscious strives after its—in the contemporary sense—unmoral ideal which the conscious mind tries to deny. (Jung, CW 7, p. 20)

Neurotic conflict provokes the realization of self-dividedness and the end of identification with the persona. A neurotic person experiences loss of self-control in that he/she is unable to bring actions into line with expectations and ideals. Such experiences introduce the possibility that one's own individual subjectivity (i.e., agency, coherence, continuity, and emotional arousal) is more complex and less understandable than one had previously imagined. The confusion and conflict of neurotic suffering becomes the potential path to the authentic individuation of self.

INDIVIDUATION AND DEVELOPMENTAL RESEARCH

The experience of self-division through neurotic suffering can lead, in Jung's view, to differentiation and integration of previously unconscious complexes. Research on structural development (e.g., stage theories of epistemological and ethical or moral development) now offers an illuminating backdrop to Jung's speculations about the development of self-reflexive or metacognitive processes through symbolic transformation.

Empirical evidence for a lifespan theory of personality development, as the typical unfolding of a human personality, was not available during Jung's lifetime. Such evidence is still largely unavailable, although we are beginning to understand some results from longitudinal studies such as those reported by Schaie (1983). As Costa, McCrae, and Arenberg (1983) report in their chapter on personality and aging, the work of Jung and Erikson, and more recently, of Gould (1978) and Levinson (Levinson, Darrow, Klein, Levinson, & McKee, 1978) has represented "the major theorizing" in the field of personality and aging (p. 222).

The results of 10 years of studies by Costa et al. on the effects of personality (measured especially by the 16PF) on aging in men are reported as contradicting the Jungian theory of individuation. As the authors state it, ". . . a Jungian theorist might even hypothesize that those apparently best adjusted in early adulthood might have the most difficult readjustment at midlife," and their results refuted this hypothetical position. Their research results are summarized as follows:

> Using the 16PF data collected 10 years previously, we showed significant positive correlations between the (Mid-Life Crisis) scale and each of the five scales loading on the General Anxiety or Neuroticism cluster. Individuals who will one day experience something that is phenomenologically similar to a mid-life crisis are those with a long history of maladjustment. . . . these longitudinal data provide compelling evidence that the mid-life crisis is more a matter of neuroticism than of development. (p. 258)

Although the authors consider these results to be in contrast with Jung's theory of individuation, they actually support it. Neurosis opens the door to midlife crisis. Neurosis invites the breakdown of the persona. In successful development, neurosis opens the door to increased insight about oneself, through psychotherapy or other relationships. Obviously, neurosis does not guarantee further development. The ability to cope with a neurosis, to seek help, and to learn from it, depends on many factors that are still not well understood.

Other researchers such as Golan (1986) and Simos (1979) connect the experience of shocking losses in midlife with the potential for reorganization of habits and attitudes that have previously been barriers to development. The cognitive and constructivist research of Loevinger (1976), Perry (1970), Belenky, Clinchy, Goldberger, and Tarule (1987), and others investigates the changing forms of thought that constitute adolescent and adult world views. These cognitive models characterize individuation as a developmental continuum of shifting attitudes about the meaning of things. The structural or stage developmental studies, in particular, support the idea of a universal development of subjectivity that is consistent with Jung's concept of a unifying self as the underlying design of an individual personality.

Only some adults continue to develop after they reach maturity. One feature they may have in common is coping with neuroticism. Coping with neuroticism means seeking help from psychotherapy, education, or religion to change. Coping with neuroticism indicates a range and strength in personal functioning that are evidence of an awareness of inner conflict, and the flexibility to respond imaginatively to oneself and one's environment. Merely enacting neuroticism usually results in loss: loss of intimate relationships, failures at work, and rigidified defenses that prevent new experiences.

Jung's perspective on the development of self emphasizes the importance of individual differences or nonnormative influences. Jung assumed that these differences become increasingly significant as a person ages. In other words, as Thurnher (1983) discovered in studying aging and ego processes, the *meaning* assigned by a person to an event, such as the loss of a parent, is more critical to the effect of the event than either the event itself or the age of the person.

The importance of individual differences in the relationship between cognitive functioning and aging is central also in predicting decreases in functioning with age, according to the results of the Seattle Longitudinal Study, as reported by Schaie (1983): "it appears that a flexible personality style in mid-life tends to predict a high level of performance in old age" (p. 129). The attitudinal differences that contribute to rigid or flexible personality styles are described by Jung in terms of the intrapsychic balancing of conscious and unconscious functions. This balancing is predicated on the breakdown or analysis of the persona.

This balancing depends on self-reflection and then on integration of psychological complexes. Those adults who make a successful transition to self-awareness have some choice in the meanings they assign to the losses and limitations of aging. Those who remain neurotically unbalanced or concretely identified with the persona tend to experience aging and dying with greater distress, both physically and psychologically.

COLLECTIVE UNCONSCIOUS, PRIMORDIAL IMAGES, AND UNITY

Jung observed a typical process or sequence of events in the achievement of a consciously integrated and differentiated personality in the second half of life. Jung's clinical evidence for this construct came from analytical work in which the analysand had differentiated the persona and the parental complexes from the self. Jung says,

> As soon as we speak of the collective unconscious we find ourselves in a sphere, and concerned with a problem, which is altogether precluded in the practical analysis of younger people or of those who have remained infantile too long. Wherever the father and mother imagos have still to be overcome, wherever there is a little bit of life still to be conquered . . . we had better make no mention of the collective unconscious . . . But once the parental transferences and the youthful illusions have been mastered, or are at least ripe for mastery, then we must speak of these things. We are here outside the range of Freudian and Adlerian reductions. . . . (CW 7, p. 74)

Jung deduced an apparently innate desire for purposive meaning (beyond the "pleasure principle," so to speak) from the lives of patients, himself, cross-cultural studies, and other biographical sources (such as dream series made available to him).

It was in his 1917 essay "On the Psychology of the Unconscious" (CW 7) that Jung first introduced the two "dominants" of unconscious structure: personal and collective. The personal unconscious was said to be organized by "memories, painful ideas that are repressed (i.e., forgotten on purpose), subliminal perceptions, by which are meant sense perceptions that were not strong enough to reach consciousness, and finally, contents that are not yet ripe for consciousness" (CW 7, p. 66).

The collective unconscious was organized by "primordial images" that are "the most ancient and the most universal 'thought-forms' of humanity" (p. 66). The primoridal images were "as much feelings as thoughts," and they led their own independent lives "rather in the manner of part-souls" (p. 66). In 1917, Jung spoke of the primordial image as the "object which the libido chooses when it is freed from the personal, infantile form of transference," revealing an unconscious organization that is not provided through experience.

It was Jung's original clinical work and research with psychotic patients at the City Hospital of Zurich that led him to posit a primordial image. From uneducated and naive patients he collected delusional images and ideas whose structure or form he found to be analogous to symbolic representations from world religions and mythologies. He relates some details from these cases in *Symbols of Transformation* (CW 5), originally published in 1916. The correspondences between dreams and fantasies of uneducated patients and the symbolic structure of mythologies prompted Jung to speculate about a collective or shared origin of symbolic form in the patterning of human development.

The central image of orderly development over the lifespan Jung called the "self" and found it was expressed in the symbol of a circle or mandala and/or a square or cross (of equal sides). Jung noted that such symbols arise spontaneously in dreams and fantasies during great psychological distress and among actively psychotic people. He believed that the figures were an unconscious attempt to impose a new order, an inherent organization, on the whole personality.

Jung also identified at that time (1916–1928) the process of compensation or balance through which unconscious images emerge to compensate conscious distortions and difficulties. An individual's ability to find meaning in self representations would depend both on motivation and on previous understanding of the persona and parental complexes.

In contemporary culture we have come to doubt the usefulness of intuitively apprehended symbols. In 1929 Jung described in a letter a kind of unconscious thought he called "apperceptive thinking" (Jung 1973b, p. 61), saying that this form of thought has "greater meaning and value" than rational thinking because it allows us to express symbols that we do not yet understand rationally. In Jung's early work, a preset or given Self (sometimes capitalized by later Jungians) is considered to be directly expressed in forms that depict a central organization of the personality, such as the circle.

The symbolic evolution of the image of the self is the factor Jung calls "God" in his formulation of apperceptive thinking. Physicist Dyson (1987) also calls this factor "God" in his formulation of theoretical physics. Like Jung, Dyson disclaims any specific theology. Dyson's account of God is similar in form and meaning to Jung's account of the self as a principle of totality:

> God is neither omniscient nor omnipotent. He learns and grows as the universe unfolds. I do not pretend to understand the theological subtleties to which this doctrine leads if one analyzes it in detail. I merely find it congenial, and consistent with scientific common sense. (Dyson, 1988, p. 119)

Jung's concept of self-formation—like Dyson's God—assumes that regulated patterns, forms, or imagination underlie experience. Intuitive apperceptions of these patterns become valid only after they have become consciously known and applied to some aspect of being.

In order for such symbolic expressions of self to be understood, or interpreted, they must be distinguished from both the material of the personal unconscious and from conscious motivations. This is possible, says Jung, only when we proceed from an assumption of final meaning, that is, the purpose we assign to an intuitively apprehended symbol after a certain amount of time has passed. When we survey long sequences of dreams and other images, and pursue their meaning in the activities of the people who experienced them, then we reason finalistically about their purpose. This can never be causal or deterministic reasoning; nor is it teleological. Rather it is backward-looking in that the interpretation is constructed only after the symbol has been known and apparently integrated into life. Jung would advise that meanings of self symbols usually cannot be understood until more than half of life is lived; otherwise we do not know the pattern or the sequence of events well enough to know the purpose of the symbol.

PSYCHOLOGICAL INDIVIDUALITY: INDIVISIBILITY

We develop psychological complexes in our early years that may or may not impede further development into authentic individuality. Jung assumes that the strong biological, sociocultural, and interpersonal patterning of infancy and early childhood results in fairly uniform development in the early years, unless there is some form of abuse or trauma. Early childhood is the "most obvious" of all periods of life from this point of view. Jung found it least interesting to study because of its greater uniformity. He did, however, develop some concepts of early childhood development, as Samuels (1985) describes. Two of Jung's most prominent followers, Neumann and Fordham, both have theories and research programs for investigating child development, but Jung himself generally deferred to Freud and Adler with few modifications.

The actual child, for Jung, is not a psychological individual. Individuation or psychological individuality demands integrity of being, an "indivisibility" that is an achievement of conscious integration of previously unconscious complexes. "Individuation means becoming an *individual*, and, in so far as *individuality* embraces our innermost, last, and incomparable uniqueness, it also implies becoming one's own self" (Jung, CW 7, p. 173).

To return then to the idea of self as an underlying form or design for the individual personality, we can now perhaps understand how Jung's self is supposed to represent the "totality" of personality. The self is a construction and expression of symbolic meanings that form a balancing or compensating relationship between conscious and unconscious life. As Jung says, "According to this definition the self is a quantity that is supraordinate to the conscious ego. It embraces not only the conscious but also the unconscious psyche, and is therefore, so to speak, a personality which we *also* are" (CW 7, p. 177).

During the early period of Jung's self theory, he believed that primordial images of the self derived from *archetypes* or original imprints of universal images. (This is a form of foundationalism similar to Kantian categories of mind.) Jung reported that adults in therapy experienced the development of self as a process that was pulling or "shaping" them, rather than one under their control. Unconscious symbolic formation was understood by Jung to be the guiding force of new development.

INFLATION AND DIFFERENTIATION

The self as a psychological center or totality was presumed to mediate the relationship between the conscious personality and unconscious complexes and images. After the persona had been analyzed and parental complexes had been understood, Jung noted a dangerous or difficult transition in analytical work and development. It was a tendency for the person to identify with the self as the center of personality. Jung describes it thus:

> The dissolution of the personality in the collective. . . . Psy-
> chologically this state is marked by a peculiar disorientation in
> regard to one's own personality; one no longer knows who one is, or
> one is absolutely certain that one actually is what one seems to have
> become. Intolerance, dogmatism, self-conceit, self-depreciation,
> and contempt for "people who have not been analysed" . . . are
> common symptoms. (CW 7, p. 282)

Jung connects this dangerous state of inflation with the beginning of a
traditional initiation ritual in which initiates have only begun to grasp a
powerful magic. Such initiations represent a psychological transition
"from the animal state to the human state" (p. 231).

In order to avoid this kind of inflated identification, Jung recommends taking a respectful and restrained attitude toward self symbolizations experienced in dreams, transference, or creative moments.
The witnessing of one's own psychic compensation, understanding the
conflict and balancing of the psyche, is a sort of testimony to meaning
and intelligence beyond one's personal will.

Jung inclines towards the notion that divinity and self are discovered to be one and the same through individuation. Recognizing an
ordering principle beyond the individual will motivates a person to
develop a dialectical relationship between psychological complexes.
One recognizes a center of personality other than the ego complex.

Jung describes initiation into self symbolization as follows: "The
individuated ego senses itself as the object of an unknown and supraordinate subject" (CW 7, p. 240). The discovery of a new perspective on
oneself results in a more objective attitude about one's own subjectivity.
Jung describes "differentiation of the self" as a "detachment of libido
from both sides," from both conscious and unconscious impulses, and
with a redirection into a broader experience of self (CW 6, p. 114). A
natural introversion results as "the libido is retained by the self and is
prevented from taking part in the conflict of opposites." The process of
differentiation and introversion results in a "detachment of disposable
libido not merely from the outer object but also from the inner object, the
thought" (CW 6, p. 115).

Through individuation in adulthood, one discovers that psychic life
is organized by opposites or polar tensions. Consciousness is always a
product of the conflict of opposites. One pole of the tension "defines" the
other, so to speak, and together they form a dynamic process of thesis
and antithesis within psychological functioning. In general, Jung's
theorizing about all aspects of personality is organized by opposites:
Eros/Logos, thinking/feeling, ego/self, personal/collective, and ex-
traversion/introversion. Eventually Jung claimed that all archetypal im-

ages are bipolar, with a positive, sustaining side, and a negative, destructive side.

INDIVIDUATION AS A DIALECTICAL PROCESS

Jung's theory of development as dialectical process assumes that the opposites are truly linked in experience; any desire to separate them always results in the "return" of the other side. As a person proceeds through the process of differentiating personal and archetypal images, complexes of one's own and those of others, and so on, the person repeatedly engages in experiences of opposites. These are experiences of suffering, a form of suffering that is different from neurotic suffering. A recognition of the necessity of suffering in life, and that human life is structured by conflict, is a central insight gained through differentiation of the self. Each renewed conflict, then, must be mediated in the same way, through a detachment of attention from either one or the other side of the pole of opposites until one can engage the "transcendent function."

This function, as we described in Chapter 1, is an individual's capacity to combine the functions of conscious and unconscious thought forms. In addition to courage, understanding, and empathy developed through individuation, a person develops "creative fantasy . . . of such a nature that it can unite the opposites. This is the function that Schiller intuitively apprehended as the source of symbols . . ." (CW 6, p. 115).

Jung's clinical descriptions of the differentiation of self and its psychological by-products are very similar to Loevinger's (1976) empirical descriptions of her later stages of ego development. Her descriptions derive from more than 30 years of research using a sentence completion test. Her last two stages of a nine-stage sequence of development emerge from what she calls the "individualistic stage" (seventh stage), marked by a heightened sense of individuality and the recognition of emotional dependence. The individualistic stage could be titled "first step of individuation," from a Jungian perspective. Loevinger describes it thus:

> The problem of dependence and independence is a recurrent one throughout development. What characterizes this level is the awareness that it is an emotional rather than a purely pragmatic problem, that one can remain emotionally dependent on others even when no longer physically or financially dependent. . . . Moralism begins to be replaced by an awareness of inner conflict. At this level, however, the conflict, for example, over marriage versus a career for a woman, is likely to be seen as only partly internal . . . That conflict is part of

the human condition is not recognized until the autonomous stage.
(1976, p. 22)

The central issue here is one of wrestling with the meaning of
conflict and dependence in the life of a mature individual. The final two
stages, autonomous and integrated, are described in Loevinger's research to include most of the themes that Jung identified in his clinical
observations. For example,

> the capacity to acknowledge and to cope with inner conflict, that is,
> conflicting needs, conflicting duties, and the conflict between needs
> and duties. . . . The autonomous person partly transcends . . .
> polarities, seeing reality as complex and multifaceted. He is able to
> unite and integrate ideas that appear as incompatible alternatives.
> . . . Self-fulfillment becomes a frequent goal, partly supplanting
> achievement. (p. 23)

And finally in Loevinger's description of the integrated stage, she adds
to her other observations the idea of a "consolidation of a sense of
identity" in the ability to deal with paradox, tolerate ambiguity, and
transcend some of the suffering of conflicts through the recognition of
their universality in human life (p. 26).

Loevinger's empirical discoveries are clearly similar to the notion of
detachment from either pole of the conflict of opposites discussed by
Jung. Loevinger depicts her sequencing of stages as a process of increasing differentiation and integration. Jung also asserts the enormous significance of differentiation for both individual and collective development of consciousness. For example,

> differentiation is a relatively late achievement of mankind, and
> presumably but a relatively small sector of the indefinitely large field
> of original identity. Differentiation is the sine qua non of conscious-
> ness. Everything unconscious is undifferentiated, and everything
> that happens unconsciously proceeds on the basis of nondifferentia-
> tion—that is to say, there is no determining whether it belongs or
> does not belong to oneself. (Jung, CW 7, p. 206)

It is remarkable that Jung's observations about the differentiation of self
and integration of unconscious complexes anticipated the constructivist
movement in psychology, and especially research on stages of ego
development. Loevinger's research findings provide empirical support
for the collective unfolding of an adult personality highly similar to that
proposed by Jung from his clinical investigations.

CONSCIOUSNESS OF SELF AS ORDER

Jung's analytical treatment proceeds largely via differentiation of psychological complexes. The analysand and analyst witness the patterns of meaning associated with symbol formation as these patterns express the conflict of opposites. Both analyst and analysand learn to resist identifying with, or projecting, any complex or any pole in the conflict of opposites, and treatment ideally proceeds via the transferential field and dreams to reveal the patterns of symbol formation. The process of learning takes place as the complexes are discharged in the transference and/or personified in dreams.

In speaking about the supraordinate powers of psychological complexes, Jung said "It is because we are not using them purposefully as functions that they remain personified complexes. So long as they are in this state, they must be accepted as relatively independent personalities" (CW 7, p. 210). The immediate goal of Jungian analysis is to reach a state in which unconscious complexes are understood in relationship to consciousness: in which a person is no longer "possessed" nor projecting but is familiar with the complexes that comprise the personality. The objective of Jungian analysis is individuation and not simply a narrative reconstruction of the past. Individuation means the recognition and acceptance of the center or the balancing of a dialectical system of "self."

This new perspective is a recognition of being organized by a center that is not synonymous with the ego complex. It is a point of view that recognizes the full character of human subjectivity, as well as the particulars of personal individuality. Jung says,

> The self could be characterized as a kind of compensation of the conflict between inside and outside. This formulation would not be unfitting, since the self has somewhat the character of a result, a goal attained, something that has come to pass very gradually and is experienced with much travail. So too the self is our life's goal, for it is the completest expression of that fateful combination we call individuality, the full flowering not only of the single individual, but of the group, in which each adds his portion to the whole. (CW 7, p. 240)

Jung's early theory of self presents both a goal and a method of development towards a more complete subjectivity of conscious and unconscious meanings and motives. Moreover, Jung opens the way to later developmental theories that trace the process of differentiation through cognitive and affective themes.

In his early theory, Jung discovers the theme of differentiation in analysis of the neuroses. He is farsighted enough to assume that neurosis may express the very urge to self-understanding that leads us into a new psychology in the late 20th century. Analysis of neuroses in the second half of life was the fertile soil in which Jung's original ideas about universal aspects of subjectivity grew. The next chapter presents aspects of Jung's broader theory of subjectivity that form a link between his early ideas about self as organizing principle and his later constructivist theories of collective mind.

☆ 4 ☆

Pattern Explanation
and Symbolic Meaning

Perhaps what characterizes Jung's self psychology more than any other single feature is his desire to explain self development in terms of acausal patterns. These explanations are indeed abstract universals, and they acquire their meaning only in context. Werner's or Piaget's developmental theories, or Chomsky's linguistic theory, and many varieties of object relations theory are other examples of pattern explanation in the human sciences. The overarching framework of pattern explanation characterizes much of Jung's theorizing about self, both in its early forms of individuality and in its later collective orientation.

Bridging the gap between the individual and collective orientations in Jung's work are several essays that depict a constructivist theory of metaphor, motivation, and development. Although we could have included other papers in this review, the essays on which we have primarily drawn are "On psychic energy" (1928/1969, CW8), "The transcendent function" (1916/1969, CW8), and "Analytical psychology and *Weltanschauung*" (1928/1969, CW8). We consider these to provide a critical sampling of Jungian idioms for a constructivist epistemology of self.

The essays and monographs that we discuss here introduce us to the broad sweep of Jung's explanations of self as a subjective experience of archetypal meaning and as an ordering principle of development.

SYMBOLS AND INSTINCTS

Jung's early work on self psychology provides a picture of individual development. In his later self psychology, especially after 1944, he shifts his attention to the collective fate of humankind and the psychology of universals: the interface between instinct and symbol. Instinct here means certain predispositions or patterned responses of behavior and affect that are inherent in human relationships (e.g., attachment routines). Symbol refers essentially to the image-making capacity of the psyche, the capacity to capture emotional meaning in visual, aural, kinesthetic, and tactile forms. The distinction between a linguistic "sign" and a "symbol," from Jung's point of view, is that a sign has a simple reference or set of references, whereas a symbol points to or indicates multidetermined meanings.

In a recent essay on the effects of "modern psychology" on Freudian theory, Helen Block Lewis (1988) stresses that many ideas and perspectives now available to psychologists were not available to Freud. She emphasizes especially the cultural nature of persons, the significance of relationships for human development, and the natural functions of dreams. "What Freud adopted as his base of theorizing was the most forward-looking materialist concept of his time: The Darwinian concept of individual instincts as the driving force in adaptation to life" (p. 8). That Freud was a biological realist is explained by Lewis as a product of the *Weltanschauung* of his time. Remarkably, Jung, writing in roughly the same period, avoids many of the pitfalls of biological reductionism. It seems to us that Jung's "comparative approach" to psychological studies, using mythology, art, and religion, resulted in pattern explanation and an appreciation of the complexity of symbolization in human life. Jung developed a method of reading the psyche through comparative patterns of symbol formation, a method analogous to modern hermeneutic psychology.

Best known perhaps of the major differences between Jung and Freud is their disagreement about the nature of libido or psychic energy. From Jung's first encounters with Freud until the end of their relationship, he refused to believe that human instincts could be reduced to a single drive, the sex drive. Eventually this refusal cost him his membership in the Viennese psychoanalytic circle. Jung assumed that instincts in humans were diverse and concerned especially with our capacity to organize unified psychic images, the foundation of symbolic representation. From the perspectives of many contemporary affect and linguistic theories, we might now judge Jung's steadfast position on the diversity and complexity of human instincts to be prescient. Of Freud's instinct theory, Lewis (1988) says,

> Freud, basing himself on a sexual instinct, assumed that faulty sexual development has a negative effect on ego development. We now know that there is indeed a linkage, but that the statement is

better turned upside down: Faulty ego development, that is, social development, has a negative effect on sexual behavior. Sexual behavior, as well as curiosity, learning skills, and many other . . . behaviors are rooted in a matrix of social relationships. (p. 13)

Jung's theory of archetype encompasses both motivational and symbolizing functions. His idea of human instinct links the archetype (as disposition to form an image) with human relationship (as the "situational pattern" in which the archetype is activated). Jungian theorists and practitioners can easily shift back and forth between an interpersonal and an intrapsychic understanding of instinct. Jung's later theory especially was affected by ethological and biological investigations of the "innate releasing mechanisms" or instinctual "programs" that contribute importantly to interpersonal patterns between people at all stages of development.

Jung assumed that the matrix of social relationship was *culture*, in the sense of the enduring symbolic representations recorded and passed down within social groups. Interfacing between culture and instinct is image. Psychological images arising in dreams and in emotionally charged moments of waking life are metaphoric models that map early interpersonal/intrapsychic experiences onto later interpersonal/intrapsychic experiences. Some of these metaphoric models will be consistent across cultures. These forms correspond to basic images of instincts such as attachment, curiosity, sexuality, and morality.

Jung used the term "psychic energy" to refer to motivation, attention, or interest in a general way, whether conscious of unconscious. Jung asserted that psychic energy transformation was always a matter of symbolic meaning, of shifts from one kind of mapping to another. Through ritual, ceremony, and mythology people transform their instinctual impulses into symbolic meanings. The symbolic transformation of psychic energy is the link between instinct and culture. As Campbell (1968) says of the "monomyth" of separation–initiation–return, the mythological adventure of the hero is "a magnification of the formula represented in the rites of passage" (p. 30). The heroic adventure into the supernatural, the encounter and conquering of fabulous forces, and the return of the hero to bestow new knowledge or prizes on others, these are the models for breaking through the parental complexes of childhood. In human life, Jung avers, symbol and instinct are inexorably related.

In her essay on Freud, Lewis (1988) reminds us that only since the influence of modern anthropology have we seen people as primarily cultural beings. She says, "Culture has many facets, but one of its universals is that human beings are organized into a society governed by moral law . . . moral law is imminent in culture and thus in human nature which develops within a society" (p. 12). The primacy of morality within human groups is in conflict with Freud's position that primitive instinctual forces must be "tamed" anew within each individual and that basic drives for self-preservation have to be converted and repressed in order to live peacefully among our kind. Freud's model of a "superego" as a parental introject is his primary concept of moral development. The superego, or the earlier version of "censorship," serves the purpose of converting the originally primitive sensual and sexual impulses into cultural aims such as learning, helping, concentrating, etc.

Jung's theory of symbolic transformation of instincts is the foundation for his assertion that morality is innate among humans. Jung believed that the transformation of instinctual impulses into moral aims is a natural or expectable development. In other words, the movement from impulse to symbol is a "moral" development, in his view. Jung believed that it was inherent in human instinctual patterns to develop a morality of reciprocity and trust with others. Although Jung had nothing like our contemporary data from ethological and infant studies, he observed many times over in his own encounters with children and others that conscience must precede guilt. He could not give an adequate explanation for what he took to be a fact, but he assumed that it was connected to the symbolizing function.

Now that we recognize the role of attachment in human behavior, we can attribute "primary altruism" to the infant's ability to relate and respond to the needs and feelings of its caregivers. Theorists such as Stern (1985), Gilligan (1982), and Belenky et al. (1986), developmental researchers such as Sroufe and Fleeson (1986), and others have concluded that the desire to provide care for others can be understood as fundamental to human nature. Traumatic and abusive experiences may interfere with the development of empathic motivation, but altruistic desires can be observed even in the earliest bonding relationship.

The function of culture, as expressed through family and society, is to initiate the individual into the transformative symbols, the metaphoric and metonymic models of self, that will provide useful and humane transitions from one to another experience of subjectivity throughout the lifespan. Every culture has a moral code that provides models for growing up and becoming a functional member of society: for initiation into adulthood, marriage, parenting, loss, grief, and death. *Moral* codes are more than rules; they are *methods* for symbolic transformation. For example, an incest taboo between brother and sister might be backed by *rules* for separating them after the age of 7 and practices for conducting business between them if they come face to face. Its main effect, however, is to transform the desire for the Other into exogamous attachments. When people live unself-consciously within the rituals of culture, they are transformed by such codes through the various ceremonies and symbolic meanings of transition.

PSYCHIC ENERGY AND TRANSFORMATION

How can we claim that Jung is a constructivist when he uses an explanatory principle such as that of psychic energy? Most explanations that rest on energic principles are materialistic, mechanistic, or realistic, claiming that truth is revealed through noninterpretive "facts" of experience. Psychic energy has never been measured or identified as different from physical energy; most contemporary psychologists consider the concept to be anachronistic and useless. Moreover, they connect it with a tradition that contrasts sharply with constructivism.

Although Jung used the idea of psychic energy sometimes in a way that might be considered as anachronistic now, he was careful to make a formal specification that identified his use as metaphorical rather than literal. In his 1928 essay on psychic energy, Jung quotes himself from a 1913 paper saying, "the libido with which we operate is not only not concrete or known, but is a complete X, a pure hypothesis, a model or counter . . ." (CW 8, p. 30).

Jung was aware of the inferential or metaphorical nature of psychic energy. His explanation of psychic energy can now be understood as "pattern explanation" (Overton, 1990). Overton gives the following description of pattern explanation:

> It introduces order and organization in the domain under investigation. Structure [or pattern, form, system, or organization—all used interchangeably here] is not directly observable and cannot . . . be reduced to observables; but . . . the method of inference is not induction but retroduction. And as a retroductive inference, pattern depends as much upon the creative internal sources of the scientist as upon the external source of observation. (p. 27)

Examples of pattern explanation in the sciences are the structure of DNA, the structure of the solar system, and the structure of the atom. Jung's explanation of psychic energy is a perfect example of a pattern explanation; in Overton's terms: "The idea of energy is not that of a substance moved in space; it is a concept abstracted from relations of movement" (Jung, CW 8, p. 4).

The energetic explanation is derived from what Jung calls a "finalistic" premise: "the event is traced back from effect to cause on the

assumption that some kind of energy underlies the changes in phenomena" (CW 8, p. 4). As we described earlier, finalistic interpretations
are *inferred* by an observer looking back over a sequence or pattern of
events, and concluding that this arrangement "makes sense" in terms of
some kind of connection to meaning. Jung uses the term "finalistic"
rather than "teleological" to avoid a misunderstanding that certain actions or events contain "the idea of an anticipated end or goal" (CW 8,
fn. 4).

Jung describes a series of hypothetical events *a*, *b*, *c*, and *d* that
develop in sequence as related in the following way: " . . . *a–b–c* are
means towards the transformation of energy, which flows causelessly
from *a*, the improbable state, entropically to *b–c*, and so on to the
probable state *d*" (CW 8, p. 31). Only "intensities of effect" are
accounted for in such an explanation, not causes. Psychic energy is thus
a metaphor for *transformation* in which events *a*, *b*, *c*, and *d* constitute a
sequence that has moved from a less probable to a more probable state,
from the point of view of the observer.

Jung does not wholly dismiss causal or mechanistic explanations in
claiming his own finalistic or energic stance. Rather, he assumes that
causal and mechanistic reasoning are legitimate perspectives for certain
situations. He uses the example of different personality types as different
points of view that lead to different styles of reasoning and explanation.
From the point of view of a metatheory or general psychology, however,
Jung rejects causal and mechanistic explanations in favor of finalistic or
pattern explanation.

PSYCHOLOGICAL ATTITUDES AND ADAPTATION

The transformations of symbolic meaning over a lifetime can be understood, within Jung's theory of psychic energy, as a pattern of progression and regression. Progression is the assumption of an attitude that
permits the use of psychic energy in a way relevant to an immediate
desire, need, or goal. Regression is the assumption of an attitude that
does not permit the use of psychic energy to reach satisfaction. Since the
immediate context is always shifting, new attitudes are frequently demanded in order to solve the difficulties or problems that impede
satisfaction. According to Jung, progression is only intermittently possible.

An attitude here means a relatively stable perspective or point of
view from which a person depicts, defines, or constructs the data of
experience into a coherent gestalt. An attitude may also be considered a
relatively stable or fixed set of assumptions that a person brings to an

experience. In the terms we borrowed earlier from Lakoff (1987), we could say also that an attitude is a propositional or image-schematic model; sometimes it may be a metaphoric or metonymic model, but usually it is the propositional or image-type model.

We will not review Jung's theory of attitudinal–functional types (CW 6)—his psychological typology—but we note that his type theory interfaces with his theory of psychic energy in the idea of "adaptation." Each Jungian type (of 16 types) is an adaptation of psychic energy use. To use Piaget's terms, a healthy person usually assimilates new experiences to already structured models of self/other that permit optimal agency, continuity, coherence, and arousal. A healthy person only accommodates to include new experiences when ongoing models or attitudes won't work or break down. If a person's attitude is too rigidly or defensively structured, however, the person will not be able to accommodate to any new or wholly different circumstances and so will tend to use the same old model even when it does not account for new experiences.

At the point that new solutions are needed in order to reach new adaptation, a rigid or strongly defended person appears to be "stopped dead," drained of energy or motivation. According to Jung, such an impasse depicts a condition in which there is an organized unconscious attitude that opposes the (habitual) conscious attitude. The longer a person remains at such an impasse, the greater the amount of associational material that gathers both around the conscious and the unconscious attitudes. This gathering of associations leads to an overwhelming sense of disunion or psychic conflict. "The stage is then set for a neurosis. The acts that follow from such a condition are uncoordinated, sometimes pathological, having the appearance of symptomatic actions" (CW 8, p. 33).

Unable to coordinate intention and action, a person feels unable to be an agent. In everyday language, we might say that the person appears to be "drained." The psychic energy that would have been directed into personal agency is used instead to activate unconscious ideas, images, and metaphors that lead into "another world," to models or meanings that are usually opposed to conscious values. "It is natural that the conscious mind should fight against accepting the regressive contents, yet it is finally compelled by the impossibility of further progress to submit to the regressive values. In other words, regression leads to the necessity of adapting to the inner world of the psyche" (CW 8, p. 36).

Jung asserts that the current conscious attitude (models for self, others, and worlds) is always balanced by unconscious attitudes that may be less adaptive at the moment but provide alternatives to consciousness. In times of unresolvable dilemmas and impasse, the unconscious models are "illuminated" and emerge more vividly in dreams and imagination. Rather than being able to use these unconscious models, either as metaphors or as alternatives for action, a person in such a state feels "captured" by them in fantasy, as images, voices, or impulses. Jung does not view this "regression" always as a "backwards development," but often as " . . . a necessary phase of development." Also he adds that "[p]rogression should not be confused with *development*" because it represents only the continuing flow of life, not necessarily differentiation (CW 8, p. 37). Progression, here, means active agency, which may be assimilation to old models and not change per se.

Only new symbolic meaning that is assigned to experiences can constitute true "development" or a change in adaptive attitude. Symbolic meaning is the ability to use a mental category to link personal experiences with collective meaning and context. One feels connected to meaning or purpose beyond oneself. From Jung's perspective, development is neither the accumulation of new experiences nor the maturation of the personality; it is always a new configuration of *meaning* with new implications for one's worldview.

MYTH AND METAPHOR: UNKNOWN WORLDS

> We construct many realities, and do so from differing intentions. But we do not construct them out of Rorschach blots, but out of the myriad forms in which we structure experience—whether the experience of the senses . . . the deeply symbolically encoded experience we gain through interacting with our social world, or the vicarious experience we achieve in the act of reading. (Bruner, 1986, p. 158)

Jung believes that the illumination of unknown worlds, of unconscious models produced from experiences lying outside ordinary awareness, introduces myth to humankind.

> We can see almost daily in our patients how mythical fantasies arise: they are not thought up, but present themselves as images or chains of ideas that force their way out of the unconscious, and when they are recounted they often have the character of connected episodes resembling mythical dramas. (CW 8, p. 38)

Myth provides the structure for culture. Essential human social and emotional expressions—innate bonding, aggression, grieving, and other patterns—are the origins of mythological images. The metaphoric language of myth is symbol. The psychological symbol, emerging wholecloth from unconscious thought processes, is the unit of expression that communicates culture to human beings, in Jung's view. Symbols arise spontaneously in dreams, creative expressions, and relationships; they are the focus of much of Jung's investigation of psychological development. "The psychological mechanism that transforms energy is the symbol" says Jung (CW 8, p. 47).

Lakoff (1987) makes a similar claim for metaphor when he says that the *conceptualizing capacity* is "The ability to form symbolic structures that correlate with *preconceptual* structures in our everyday experience. Such symbolic structures are basic-level and image-schematic concepts" (p. 281). Both Jung and Lakoff presume that unconscious thought organizes the development of symbolic meaning in culture.

As we alluded to earlier, Jung defines "symbol" as a representational image that is "alive" or motivating for a person; he contrasts this to "sign," which is verbal, digital, a pointer or a signal. Whereas a symbol generates new meaning by mapping experiences in a new domain, a sign only signals that something is so within an already-established system. For example, for many Americans, the symbol of "sacrifice" is alive in personal, social, and cultural domains generating fresh meanings in regard to such "modern" forms of suffering as AIDS, child sexual abuse, and Holocaust survival. On the other hand, the "sign of the cross" is primarily a signal in contemporary American life, pointing to a form of Christianity. Once it might have been a living symbol, but now for many people, it is a sign. Whether a particular image, gesture, event, or ritual is symbol or sign depends on the personal context, the attitude of the observer or person.

Symbols should be interpreted analogically or metaphorically (not translated literally), according to Jung, in terms of their mythic meanings, working to and fro between different experiential domains. Signs, on the other hand, are to be translated literally or rationally, in terms of propositional or image-schematic models.

Jung's idea of symbol is of a working metaphor whose meaning is revealed through living. Consequently, Jung insists on interpreting *sequences* of dreams, rather than a single dream, and in coming to understand the meaning of a psychological *symptom* (which he considers to be a purposive symbol rather than a sign of disease) over time. This is a finalistic method of interpretation, the self-conscious "backwards glance" in which the purpose of the symbol may be constructed from lived experiences as they are remembered.

Jung deemphasizes the development of reasoning and abstract thought in his psychology in favor of understanding metaphorical schemata that are depicted in mythological and artistic motifs. Metaphorical schemata, or mythological thinking, originate in instinctual expressions organized as *situational patterns* and communicated through human relationship. Mythological meaning depicts the symbolic transformations of human beings over the lifespan from birth to death.

Human emotions are organized systems of arousal and expression. Positive emotions (such as joy and interest/excitement) and negative emotions (such as sadness, anger, fear, and shame) are recognized universally to have particular meanings. Researchers such as Tomkins (1962, 1987) and Izard (1977) have investigated the meanings of emotional expressions in literate and other societies. Their results strongly suggest the existence of unconscious structures or patterns that shape the expression of affective-imaginal life among humans.

Jung does not entirely reject a reductive sign-oriented interpretation of symbols, such as an explanation of symptoms (considered to be symbols) as infantile impulses, but he assumes that such an interpretation is incomplete and sometimes misleading. Jung returns always to the purposive nature of symbols as intelligence revealed from unconscious sources. The major function of symbols is culture-making, expressing the link between instinct or embodiment and the symbolic world. Repeatedly Jung emphasizes the following:

> The contents of the collective unconscious are . . . the results of the psychic functioning of our whole ancestry; in their totality, they compose a natural world-image, the condensation of millions of years of human experience. These images are mythological and therefore symbolical, for they express the harmony of the experiencing subject with the object experienced. All mythology and all revelation come from this matrix of experience, and all our future ideas about the world and man will come from it likewise. (CW 8, p. 380)

Much of our mental experience, Jung contends, is not ever conscious at all; thoughts arrive, and we have access to them but not to their productive processes.

Individual symbol production, especially through inspiration, dreams, and fantasy life, gives each person access to images of self-construction and reconstruction, especially at critical points in the lifespan. As Jung says, modern individuals especially need to be alert to affect-laden symbols because symbols allow us to use our energies for "effective work." Without symbolic connections we lack motivation to create ourselves and to foster the conditions of our own development.

> Only where a symbol offers a steeper gradient than nature is it possible to canalize libido into other forms. The history of civilization has amply demonstrated that man possesses a relative surplus of energy that is capable of application apart from the natural flow. (CW 8, p. 47)

Modern and postmodern cultures offer little in the way of initiation into symbolic life. In a lecture given by Jung in 1939 (CW 18, pp. 267–290), he relates a conversation he had had with "the master of ceremonies" of a tribe of Pueblo Indians, contrasting the traditional symbolic life of Native Americans with the individualism of modern American society. At a critical moment, the master of ceremonies says,

> "Now look at these Americans: they are always seeking something. They are always full of unrest, always looking for something. What are they looking for? There is nothing to be looked for!" (p. 275)

And Jung responds,

> That is perfectly true. You can see them, these travelling tourists, always looking for something, always in the vain hope of finding something. . . . I met a woman in Central Africa who had come up alone in a car from Cape Town and wanted to go to Cairo. "What for?" I asked . . . And I was amazed when I looked into her eyes—the eyes of a hunted, a cornered animal. . . . She is nearly possessed; she is possessed by so many devils that chase her around. And why is she possessed? Because she does not live the life that makes sense. (p. 275)

Without the means of translating mythological images into personal meaning, many people lack the ability to sustain a symbolic life. Traditional cultures provide the means for all members to learn the language of myth and to translate their dream images and personal longings into a bigger picture of human purpose.

Jung points especially to puberty rites and initiation ceremonies as the introduction to living the symbolic life. The young-adult initiate is separated from the parents "by magical means." The ceremony is not only a separation from the actual parents, but it is an induction into adult symbols and meanings. For this transition to take place, each young person must account for what is lost or rejected from childhood. Jung calls this the "injured" parental archetype.

> There must be no more longing backward glances at childhood, and for this it is necessary that the claims of the injured archetype should be met. This is done by substituting for the intimate relationship with the parents another relationship, namely that with the clan or tribe. The infliction of certain marks on the body, such as circumcision and scars, is intended to serve this end, as also the mystical instruction which the young man receives during his initiation. (CW 8, p. 374)

Jung points out that simply parting from one's actual parents is "not sufficient" because such a separation lacks the notion of *sacrifice* or of surrendering to powers larger than oneself. Initiation ceremonies teach the initiate to "act against nature" and learn the lesson of consciousness so as not to become the victim of impulses, wishes, and infantile longings. "This is indeed the beginning of all culture, the inevitable result of consciousness and of the possibility of deviating from unconscious law" (CW 8, p. 375).

Symbolic meaning in Jung's psychology involves both the idea that emergent metaphors "make sense" through living (in coming to know the meaning of archetypal patterns), and the notion that living symbols cannot be reduced to discrete categories or rational formulas. Critical of Freud's "monomyth" of infantile sexuality as the central motivator for symptoms, art, myth, and culture, Jung maintains a distinction between *emergent meaning* as "living symbol" (in myth, art, and religion) and *infantile complexes* as repetitive compulsions motivated by sexual impulses or other wishes and fears.

In his 1916 essay "The Transcendent Function" (CW 8), Jung emphasizes especially the influence of living symbols on the development of self. Living symbols inspire affect and action in the people who experience them. The ability to understand living symbols depends on cultivating a particular psychological function that Jung calls "transcendent" because it permits an observing attitude that "transcends" polarities of conscious/unconscious, good/bad, and right/wrong. This attitude occurs naturally, especially at critical turning points throughout the lifespan, but must be strengthened and developed if a person is to live a conscious life. A conscious life is one in which both sides of a conflict can be perceived and understood from an "objective" third position.

In order to cultivate this attitude, Jung recommends a "constructive" or "synthetic" method of interpretation of living symbols (e.g., from dreams and the transferential field) to stand alongside the "reductive" or "analytic" method. The constructive method is not to replace the analytic, but to accompany it. The constructive method is the work of expanding the meaning of an image or symbol in order to discover its *purpose in the moment*. It answers the question "Why at this moment does this symbol arise?" The analytic method is the work of reducing the meaning of an image or symbol in order to discover its *source, cause, or history* within the life of the individual. It answers the question "From what does this symbol originate?"

A living symbol has a certain "surprise" or alien character that generates inspiration and instigates action. When using the constructive method, Jung first gathers a person's own associations to a symbol or image, but not to use them simply to formulate an explanation, even to answer the question "Why do you produce this?" Rather, he uses them as a background to which are added new and unfamiliar meanings—references to cultural forms: traditional mythologies, religions, folklore, or artistic expressions. In this way a dream image or a transferential "moment" can be expanded into a world of meaning that may open a new vista or purpose. For instance, an image of a talking serpent might be associated personally with experiences of sudden fright, exotic power, and distressing childhood memories. A Jungian "synthesis" of these associations with similar images and metaphors from mythology, art, literature, or religion provides a new construction of the meaning of a talking serpent. The new construction might include references to the divine serpents of oracular wisdom, the association of serpents with healing, the motifs of transformation using the serpent metaphor (shedding skin and rebirth), or connection of the serpent with the Great Mother or Goddess ceremonies. The constructive method often reveals a purpose or an intelligence in the occurrence of the symbol that goes beyond what was consciously known.

The constructive or synthetic method is "analogical" rather than "logical." Analogical means "pattern recognition" or the method of expanding knowledge through comparisons. The synthetic method involves the use of mythologems to expand from one pattern to another of similar structure. The synthetic method explores *emotional purposes* expressed in metaphors or living symbols, but it does not diagnose the causes or antecedents, such as historical meanings. Any particular symbol or imagistic expression may be interpreted as universal (analogical) or personal (logical, related to the affective particulars of a psychological complex) or both. To consider only the personal, historical meaning is inadequate to understanding the full psychological function of symbolic expression, according to Jung.

The development of the transcendent function, as an attitude of waiting and exploring both purpose and cause, is a central goal in Jungian analysis. In Bruner's (1986) discussion of emotional meaning, he says "Emotion is not usefully isolated from knowledge of the situation that arouses it. Cognition is not a form of pure knowing to which emotion is added. . . . And action is a final common path based on what one knows and feels" (p. 118). Jung's essay on the transcendent function traces a useful method for reuniting emotion, cognition, and action through interpreting living symbols as metaphors that emerge from our immediate contact with the field of universal being. Opening the door to many worlds of meaning is the intention we read in Jung's treatment of psychological disturbances. Engendering or encouraging the transcendent function, through the use of both synthetic and analytic methods, is a primary curative factor in Jungian analysis.

The transcendent function increases a person's ability to shuttle "to and fro" between the universal and the personal, coping with ambiguity, tolerating paradox, synthesizing opposites. In the best constructivist tradition, Jung advocated relativism of psychological worlds:

> One of the greatest obstacles to psychological understanding is the inquisitive desire to know whether the psychological factor adduced is "true" or "correct." If the description of it is not erroneous or false, then the factor is valid in itself and proves its validity by its very existence. (CW 8, p. 91)

WELTANSCHAUUNG AND SELF

> The man whose sun still moves round the earth is essentially different from the man whose earth is a satellite of the sun. . . . The man whose cosmos hangs in the empyrean is different from one whose mind is illuminated by Kepler's vision. The man who is still dubious about the sum of twice two is different from the thinker for whom nothing is less doubtful than the a priori truths of mathematics. In short, it is not a matter of indifference what sort of *Weltanschauung* we possess, since not only do we create a picture of the world, but this picture changes us. (CW 8, pp. 361–362)

Jung parallels *Weltanschauung* with folk wisdom or common sense when he says that it comprises a person's best efforts to be objective and unopinionated in establishing a picture of the world "as it is." In contemporary Western societies this picture includes the knowledge that "knowledge is limited and subject to error" (CW 8, p. 362). Because we are aware that we grasp the world as a psychic image, when the image of the world changes, we cannot tell whether the world has changed or we have changed.

Our awareness of the recursive process of world construction frees our imagination to develop the transcendent function. According to Jung: "Every new discovery, every new thought, can put a new face on the world. We must be prepared for this, else we suddenly find ourselves in an antiquated world, itself a relic of lower levels of consciousness" (CW 8, p. 363).

One example of such a relic, according to Jung, is the psychoanalytic world view. In Freudian theory, one is faced with a rational materialism of the late 19th century, grounded in an antiquated form of reductionism. No other picture and no other form of thought can be derived from this form of psychoanalytic interpretation: the aim of interpretation is to bring instinctual motivations to consciousness and make repression unnecessary by conscious correction. Meaning is fixed as biological realism or rationalism that precludes the creativity of unconscious thought.

If psychoanalysis offers such a narrow world view why is it compelling to so many? Jung says it is because of the "devastation" that has been wrought by repressions and our ignorance of instinctual processes:

> There is no form of human tragedy that does not in some measure proceed from this conflict between the ego and the unconscious. Anyone who has ever seen the horror of a prison, an insane asylum, or a hospital will surely experience, from the impression these things make upon him, a profound enrichment of his *Weltanschauung*. (CW 8, p. 366)

Psychoanalysis has revealed the underlying components of the conditions that feed human tragedy, and so it appears to provide relief from that tragedy. Yet psychoanalysis has not offered a new *Weltanschauung*, different from 19th-century materialism. When we reduce "a poem of Goethe's" to his "mother-complex" or "explain Napoleon" as a "case of masculine protest" or "St. Francis as a case of sexual repression," we confine ourselves to our own compulsive repetitions of reductive explanations and to an impossible psychology of the self. According to Jung

> The mistake . . . lies in the circumstance that psychoanalysis has a scientific but purely rationalistic conception of the unconscious. When we speak of instincts we imagine that we are talking about something known, but in reality we are talking about something unknown. As a matter of fact, all we know is that effects come to us from the dark sphere of the psyche which somehow or other must be assimilated into consciousness if devastating disturbances of other functions are to be avoided. (CW 8, p. 367)

Jung recommends taking an "as if" attitude toward unconscious processes, remembering that we simply act "as if" we know. Unconscious processes are in fact unknown, unavailable to our observation, and hence are more practically understood as "a great X." All infantile complexes become autonomous unconscious complexes organizing unconscious processes through their affective meanings, the archetypes. Jung assumes that these complexes are personified and projected as "spirits, demons, and gods" within a "primitive" *Weltanschauung* that considers such powers to be extrahuman. The complexes are projected onto the world. In this kind of world, these denizens must be respected and handled as powers that escape the realm of human desires and control. Within a materialist world view, on the other hand, one assumes that such powers can be defeated through a scientific or biological explanation.

One of the common ways in which infantile complexes influence us is through neurosis. Typically the neurosis is considered negligible in itself; it is merely a symptom to be eliminated through an explanation. The explanation theoretically frees a person to restore full powers to the self. Here is where Jung differs with the rationalism of psychoanalysis and sets forth his own psychological constructivism rooted in image-schematic and metaphorical models of mind.

Although the affective particulars of an individual complex can be explained in terms of infantile meanings, the universal aspects of the complex (archetypal meanings and pattern) cannot. Universal meanings connected to archetypal states can be penetrated only with respect, courage, and imagination: the transcendent function. Reductive explanations that attempt to defeat the power of the unconscious result in "[a] dissociation between conscious and unconscious . . . and then the activity of the unconscious begins. This is usually felt as very unpleasant, for it takes the form of an inner, unconscious fixation which expresses itself only symptomatically" (CW 8, p. 374). By contrast, a combination of synthetic and analytic methods fosters a differentiation and relativism of forms of thought: The recognition that dream, symptom, metaphor, and imagination are emotionally-laden images that cannot be exhaustively explained, but must be allowed to stand side by side with rational forms of thought. The collective unconscious, organized by archetypal forms

> constitutes in its totality a sort of timeless and eternal world-image which counterbalances our conscious, momentary picture of the world. It means nothing less than another world, a mirror-world if you will. But, unlike a mirror-image, the unconscious image possesses an energy peculiar to itself, independent of consciousness. (CW 8, p. 376)

Constructivist theorists assert the power of metaphoric thought as pattern recognition and comparison. Jung asserts the power of archetypal images as multidetermined, analogic, and shaped by universal affects and situational patterns. Archetypal images cannot be explained away by causal factors of individual history. Our contemporary recognition of our own capacity to create psychic realities means that we no longer live in a world infused with extrahuman powers, the gods and goddesses. Speaking to our condition, Jung cautions, "it would be a misunderstanding to suppose that the fantasy-images of the unconscious can be used directly, like a revelation. They are only the raw material, which, in order to acquire a meaning, has first to be translated into the language of the present" (CW 8, p. 380). If our translation is successful, we can have some access to an experience of universal humanness. "This is an experience which comes very close to that of the primitive, who symbolically unites himself with the totem-ancestor by partaking of the ritual feast" (CW 8, p. 380).

Claiming that myth, metaphor, and symbol may constitute a "nonanalyzable" affective-imaginal intelligence results in a new *Weltanschauung*. We understand the powers of rationality to be limited and the source of our most creative moments to be somehow beyond our control. Yet we also recognize that all of these arise from a subjective experience and not from the conditions of an objective world "out there." The *Weltanschauung* offered through Jungian methods is one that is self-consciously recursive and not reduced to rational meaning.

> A *Weltanschauung* is not made for the world, but for ourselves. If we do not fashion for ourselves a picture of the world, we do not see ourselves either, who are the faithful reflections of that world. Only when mirrored in our picture of the world can we see ourselves in the round. Only in our creative acts do we step forth into the light and see ourselves whole and complete. Never shall we put any face on the world other than our own, and we have to do this precisely in order to find ourselves. (CW 8, p. 379)

This especially constructivist explanation of *Weltanschauung* leads us into a discussion of collective mind in the terms Jung outlined in his later work. After his convalescence in 1944, and until his death in 1961, Jung labored over the idea that the unity of the world is constructed collectively in a manner that reflects the unity of the self. To put this another way, Jung assumed that investigating the process by which world and self are constructed would reveal the mysteries of both. Similar to Piaget, Jung was interested in understanding how and why the psychological construction of the physical world could reflect the "reality" of that world. How did our image of the world reveal the mind that created it or vice versa? The next chapter is our attempt to answer this question through Jung's analysis of the problem behind it.

☆5☆

Archetypal Self:
Knower and Known

The whole course of individuation is dialectical, and the so-called "end" is the confrontation of the ego with the "emptiness" of the centre. Here the limit of possible experience is reached; the ego dissolves as the reference point of cognition. It cannot coincide with the centre, otherwise we would be insensible: that is to say, the extinction of the ego is at best an endless approximation. (Jung, 1975, p. 259)

Individuation can be understood as the design for the development of individual subjectivity through an increasing ability to review the character of one's own existence, to unpack the mysteries with a sense for their meaning and purpose. This involves an ability to use the ego complex to survey the meaning of self over time.

Reflections on meaning and purpose tend to support either one or both of our experiential theories of time: linear or cyclical. Thus, people may appear to themselves to be moving through a linear sequence of events (such as childhood, youth, and maturity) or through a cycle of integrations (such as repeated encounters with attachment, separation, and loss). They may appear to themselves to be in a combination of these two experiences of time, in a "spiral" of repeating patterns that moves in an irreversible direction.

In the above quote Jung alludes to a metacognitive process in which the individual subject (the ego) increasingly finds evidence of having been organized around an "empty center": The person infers a meaningful pattern or center of life that has not been intended but has apparently been purposive. Jung considers this an experience of "being the object" of another subjectivity. This thesis, as we have said, is an "argument from design" (see Dennett, 1987.) The argument asserts that an event (a life, in this case) or configuration may be said to have an implied meaning that may never be known directly, but can be inferred from its patterns or form. Continuity, as the self developing throughout the lifespan, is inferred especially through our constructions of time.

The topic of this chapter is Jung's final conceptualization of self and its coordinates. Largely this is a design model of individuation that has been conflated with the archetype of self. Jung used the metaphor of the self to stand for both the totality (or design) of the whole personality and the experience of being an individual.

As we mentioned earlier, his theory changed substantially after 1944. Enigmatic and significant contributions to self psychology emerge from this last period of his work: (1) recognition of the archetype as pure form (archetype *an sich*); (2) the "psychoid" nature of archetypes as the interface between the psychological world and the phenomenological world of "outer" events; (3) the theory of synchronicity as a principle of "acausal" connection between events in the phenomenological world (e.g., the "accidental" stopping of a clock at a particular time) that take on meaning in regard to psychological experiences (e.g., grief related to the death of a relative at the time the clock stopped); and (4) the hierarchical organization of self through individuation, as a spiraling of patterns recursively experienced as different self-images (presented in *Aion: Researches into the Phenomenology of the Self*, CW 9, II).

These contributions appear to contrast with Jung's earlier work because they focus primarily on the fabric of collective being rather than on individual personality functioning. Our purpose is to present them in the light of contemporary constructivism, and to clarify their assumptions in a manner consistent with Jung's intentions. From this perspective, we emphasize especially the symbolic nature of time, and the nature of human embodiment and emotional arousal as they affect our perceptions of self and world.

Archeologist Gould (1987) has suggested that two basic metaphors for time, "time's arrow" and "time's cycle," are powerful schematic organizers for ordinary life and scientific theory. The metaphor of time's arrow depicts the irreversibility of a sequence of events, the inevitability of movement from beginning to middle to end. The metaphor of time's cycle, by contrast, shows an oscillating or circular repetition of pattern and organization that recurs in regular, and perhaps predictable, episodes. For our purposes, we appropriate the metaphor of time's arrow for the experience of personal subjectivity as "ego" across the lifespan. We use the image of time's cycle for the subjective recognition of Jung's "self" as organization around a center. In Gould's (1987) words, we can describe the experience of ego as "the irreversibility of history, and the unrepeatable uniqueness of each step in a sequence of events linked through time in physical connection" (p. 194). Self, by contrast, is "those aspects of nature that are either stable or else cycle in simply repeating (or oscillating) series because they are direct products of nature's timeless laws, not the contingent moments of complex historical pathways" (p. 196). In light of earlier chapters, we can translate "nature's timeless laws" as the invariants of self: agency, coherence, continuity, and emotional arousal, the conditions that constrain and engender self. These invariants are reorganized according to new demands at each new phase of the life cycle, and they reappear as the central aspects of self with new meanings.

Jung believes that the *mandala* or circular form expresses this meaning of self in Hindu, Buddhist, and Christian art and rituals in which the development of subjective truth or self-knowledge is portrayed as a "circumambulation" or a meditation on a center. Contemporary ethological and evolutionary theories of biology and psychology (e.g., Maturana & Varela, 1980) also depict knowledge development as circular or cyclical. The spiral of recursive development, the structuring of metaprocesses or thinking about thought, is a contemporary model for the development of a self-reflective subjectivity. For example, Guidano (1987) says,

> the slow unfolding of cognitive abilities makes possible awareness . . . of their presence only at a later stage, usually adolescence and early adulthood. Only at this time may the relationship between tacit and explicit knowledge undergo a reorganization . . . structured into a conscious self-image capable of actively directing the programming of one's life. (p. 23)

Because of this recursive patterning—first of matching (assimilation) and later of reorganization (accommodation)—the form of the spiral or circle has been used by developmental theorists and object relations theorists to convey the idea of "eternal return" in the rhythm of human thoughts and desires.

In constructivist theories, knowledge is recognized as a fundamental property of all complex living systems. Knowledge is not "merely conceptual" but is a method of life. Knowledge is problem solving that develops in sustained interactions between organisms and their environments. Knowledge is the building of representations from these interactions, generalized so that the models themselves can be corrected by further experience. Biologists Maturana and Varela (1980) have demonstrated that processes of pattern recognition belong to all complex living systems, not just to the higher primates and humans.

What distinguishes persons from other sentient beings is probably the fact that human pattern recognition has been extended and developed to include substantial "decentering" and abstraction. To remove ourselves from the center of our own subjectivity is to be able to see ourselves and other worlds, and, hence, to investigate other organisms and objects. Again, to quote Guidano (1987),

> With this ability to reach beyond the perceptual field, human beings attained an unprecedented level of disengagement from the immediacy of experience and acquired new possibilities to explore and control the environment, as well as an ever increasing level of comprehension of themselves and the world. (p. 18)

Our abstractions are sustained in reflection as well as in action, and are shaped into complex theories about ourselves and other worlds.

Indeed, the quote from Jung that opens this chapter suggests that we can observe ourselves as decentering from our identification with the ego or time's arrow, increasingly to experience ourselves as evolving through time's cycle, organized by a "centre" that is not directly perceivable. Thus, we decenter and infer an abstract process of self as a universal form by which all individual subjects are designed to develop.

The processes of abstraction and decentering have been investigated especially by Piaget and his followers, and by Luria (1979) and Vygotsky (1978). These are means by which people develop metacognitive abilities so that they can effectively direct and master their own cognitions, their thoughts and feelings. Through an initial process of decentering (moving out of the actual identification with the subjectivity of one's experiences), the young child organizes an identity as an individual subject. The birth and organization of this identity of self interfaces with the birth and organization of a "world." As Guidano (1987) says, "the maintenance of one's perceived identity becomes as important as life itself; without it the individual would be incapable of proper functioning and would lose . . . the very sense of reality" (p. 3).

Guidano (1987), like Lakoff (1987) and Johnson (1987), stresses the idea that embodiment is frequently the image-scheme for our basic propositional models for what we perceive as reality:

> We are three dimensional organisms, and we structure space in terms of height, width, and depth. Moreover, having a sense of self that is perceived as individuality and uniqueness, we are similarly led to consider entirely natural the ordering of reality within a set of circumscribed entities to which we attribute such individuality. (Guidano, 1987, p. 9)

Individuality and uniqueness arise through our subjective experience of separate body-being and are also perceived as existing in other body-beings, both animate and inanimate.

Why is the archetype of self, of individual subjectivity, so powerful an organizer of human life when it does not appear to be as powerful in other life forms? Jungian analyst Neumann attempted to answer this question in *The Origins and History of Consciousness* (1954). Neumann suggested that a unified individual self-image is a product of the evolutionary development and management of a complex nervous system. He used the term "centroversion" to name the process involved in the phylogenetic and phenomenological advent of selfhood in a structurally complex organism. Guidano (1987), Popper (1975), Weimer (1977, 1982), and Pribram (1980) now have made the same point. Selfhood seems to be the consequence of human embodiment, the product especially of a structurally complex organism that processes diverse forms of information and can best manage these by developing a unified image of itself.

ARCHETYPE, OBJECTIVITY, AND EPISTEMIC SUBJECT

We begin with a comparison between Jung's final formulation of self as archetype *an sich* (as such), as pure form, and Piaget's account of an "epistemic subject." Besides showing the similarity between the structural theory of these two psychologists, our comparison should illuminate some of the epistemological difficulties of the idea of an "empty center." This will lead us into Jung's elaboration of self theory in his *Answer to Job* (CW 11) and *Aion* (CW 9, II).

Writing of archetype as form, Jung emphasized a biological metaphor—the "pattern of behavior"—in which a situational action exhibits inherent intelligence that cannot have been learned. In 1955, Jung wrote of *archetype:*

> This term is not meant to denote an inherited idea, but rather an inherited mode of psychic functioning, corresponding to the inborn way in which the chick emerges from the egg, the bird builds its nest, a certain kind of wasp stings the motor ganglion of the caterpillar, and eels find their way to the Bermudas. In other words, it is a "pattern of behaviour." This aspect of the archetype, the purely biological one, is the proper concern of scientific psychology. (CW 18, p. 518)

This "ethological" definition of archetype is typical of Jung's later work, most closely related to constructivism and evolutionary theory. He frequently contrasts his ethological description of archetype with clinical or experiential descriptions of archetypal functioning encountered in psychotherapy.

Confrontation with an archetypal image in a dream or waking life is, according to Jung, "numinous"—captivating and fascinating in an awesome way. As we detailed in the last chapter, Jung calls attention to the transformative power of imagery from dreams and creative expressions in fostering transformation from one phase of the lifespan to the next. The function of archetypal images is especially apparent in myths that are used collectively to inform and make sense out of transformations over the lifespan.

Jung uses the metaphor of the "atom" to depict the archetypal organization of individual subjectivity. In this metaphor, the self is the nucleus or center that holds together the disparate but related complexes of the personality. The ego complex "rotates" around the self in a unique energy field. Other identity complexes—persona, shadow, parental complexes, and the relational complexes of anima/animus—also rotate, but they do not share the subjective power of the ego–self "axis."

Personal recognition of a center of the personality is a product of decentering or metacognition in the second half of life, as we explained in Chapter 2. Experiences of an archetypal self emerge through recognizing the transformations that permit us to move from one stage of development to the next, grounded in the invariants of our own subjectivity. Traditionally these transformations—were collectively realized through ritual and ceremony. In modern life they are often recognized only through reflections on our own and others' experiences of neuroses, dreams, emotional states, and personal distress.

In order for anyone to infer a central organizing form or design of personality, she/he must be able to *decenter*—to disidentify with the ego complex or time's arrow. Having achieved a kind of objectivity about subjective processes, such a person is able to form hypotheses about the larger patterns of meaning that can be construed in the transformations of life.

The knowledge of one's death makes this move both difficult and necessary, from Jung's point of view. The knowledge of individual extinction makes it difficult to decenter from the ego complex because of the stunning fear associated with one's own disappearance and separation from attached others. On the other hand, from Jung's viewpoint, decentering from the ego is necessary because it transforms the narcissism of early adulthood. The original identity of the ego complex with the vitality of expansion and acquisition has to be transformed into accepting the difficult fate of loss and surrender. The depression from losses connected with aging and death can defeat even the most heroic ego, and so a person must transform the heroic image of self into some other identity meaning.

Through the process of individuation and the recognition of inner conflict and compensation, a person is able to transform narcissistic losses into symbolic meaning, to transform individual suffering into a sort of "objective" curiosity about the meaning of life and fate. Jung observed that some (individuating) people live their later years far more fruitfully and pleasantly than others. Those who live most fully seem to embrace some aspect of time's cycle and the symbolism of transformation in which individual extinction can be embedded or contextualized. That is, they can decenter from their preoccupations with individual power, desire, and fear.

In a book about the evolutionary purpose of objectivity, philosopher Nagel (1986) fails to see any manner in which objectivity can be applied to one's own extinction. He says,

> The objective standpoint may try to cultivate an indifference to its own annihilation, but there will be something false about it: the individual attachment to life will force its way back even at this level. (pp. 230–231)

Nagel believes we are unable to decenter from an identification with time's arrow, and he is convinced that individual attachment to life circumvents any attempt to be objective about one's death. Otherwise careful to extol the virtues of objectivity and decentering, Nagel here is convinced that there is an irreconcilable clash between objective knowledge and one's own death. The anticipation of death makes one subjectively "small," according to Nagel, acutely identified with the ego complex.

> The objective standpoint simply cannot accommodate at its full subjective value the fact that everyone, oneself included, inevitably dies. There really is no way to eliminate the radical clash of standpoints in relation to death. (Nagel, 1986, p. 230)

Both Piaget and Jung seem to disagree with Nagel. Piaget and Jung ground their arguments in similar starting points. They do not find individual subjectivity to be a "thing in itself" or the sole access to experiences of subjectivity. Hence, a person is not so tightly bound to time's arrow or the ego complex.

Piaget, in fact, refused even to develop a theory of individual subjectivity on the grounds that his psychology was a study of universal psychological processes and not of unique subjectivity. His construct of the "epistemic subject" is clearly analogous to Jung's archetypal self in its latest (ethological) form. "The organization of subjectivity that is common to all human subjects" could be the definition of either. Broughton (1987), quoting Beth and Piaget (1966), gives the Piagetian definition of the epistemic subject as "that which all subjects have in common, since the general coordinations of actions permit a universal which is that biological organization itself" (p. 284).

Moreover, Piaget aligns this "operational self" with "God," who is "unceasingly constructing ever 'stronger' systems" (quoted in Broughton, 1987, p. 285). He assumes that there is evidence for such a central organizing principle as God in the structural invariants of human knowledge. The image-schematic model for this central organizing principle is also, for Piaget, the "center" (implying the metaphor of circle). Elaborating this idea, Piaget emphasizes the circular interactions of assimilation and accommodation that define the structure of human knowing. Throughout his work, he returns to the ideal of "decentering" as the successful goal of true development, the ability to free oneself from one's egocentrism. Decentering especially requires the ability to accommodate or to change one's previously held knowledge system, to change one's mind. According to Piaget, the process of decentering is the "true generator" of structures (in Broughton, 1987, p. 286). It is not the individual subject who is able to develop new knowledge systems, but rather it is the case that "the subject exists because, to put it very briefly, the being of structures consists in their coming to be, that is, their being 'under construction' " (Broughton, 1987, p. 286). The epistemic subject, the being of structures, is the underpinning of new knowledge systems and is "a center of activity" (Broughton, 1987, p. 286).

What is this center of activity? Broughton, in his critique of Piaget's theory of subjectivity, avers that we cannot find an answer to this question in Piaget. Broughton, wondering whether this being of structures can know itself, says that "Piaget nowhere indicates that consciousness is a characteristic of the epistemic subject. Moreover . . . he is inclined to associate consciousness with the psychological subject, and to use the concept of the epistemic subject to play down the significance of consciousness" (p. 289). Left empty of its own subjectivity and representing an abstract system of its own evolution, the epistemic subject can be abused, claims Broughton. It can be used as an organizing rationale for any institution of authority, science, or reason. If the epistemic subject has come to mean a normative structure without its own subjectivity, then it can be filled with any authoritative voice or movement.

We believe that Broughton makes an error of analysis when he attempts to interpret the "subjectivity" of the epistemic subject. The epistemic subject is a design model of subjectivity, and so cannot be interpreted from a functional or intentional stance. The "subject" here is similar to Jung's "self" of the individuation model. There is no analogy between an intentional subject and the center of a design. The idea of consciousness implies human intentionality, and Broughton assumes that the epistemic subject could be understood from an intentional perspective as we would understand the individual subject. Broughton believes that Piaget leaves open the question about intentionality of the epistemic subject, but we wonder if Broughton is raising a question on a different level of analysis from the one intended by Piaget. Whether it is Broughton or Piaget who is posing the question about consciousness in the epistemic subject, Jung provides an "answer to Piaget" in his essay about the subjectivity of the epistemic subject, a monograph called *The Answer to Job* (CW, 11).

Before turning to this material, let us look briefly again at Jung's understanding of the development of self in terms of the last period of his work. Jung suggests that we can explain the universal design of subjectivity and knowledge as "natural forces that appear in us as instincts" *or* as the "will of God" without doing injustice to his meaning either way. If we take the instinctual explanation, the position Bowlby takes in his ethological theory of attachment, there are potentially dangerous consequences for our psychological health, claims Jung. He fears we will lose touch with "our moral self-esteem" and our ability to see ourselves as part of a larger meaning system. By this, he means that if we accept a "just so" explanation of unconscious processes, then we lose the "as if" attitude that includes a sense of respect for the mystery that pervades our existence. Jung assumes that an instinctual explanation is a reductive "just so" explanation.

To explain the structure of individuation and the development of the self, Jung prefers a greater and more complex model than a person, a model more like "God" (CW 9, II, p. 27). According to Jung, if we see ourselves as the "objects" of a greater subjectivity, parts of a larger being, we can live in better harmony with the *habitus* of our "ancestral psychic life" (CW 9, II, p. 27). "So when I say that the impulses which we find in ourselves should be understood as the 'will of God,' I wish to emphasize that they ought not to be regarded as an arbitrary wishing and willing, but as absolutes which one must learn how to handle correctly" (p. 27).

Jung compares his notion of the will of God with the Greek term "daimon," which names a determining power acting on humans "like providence or fate, though the ethical decision is left to man" (p. 27). By connecting the universals of subjectivity and knowledge to the will of

God, then, Jung argues in favor of a God metaphor to fill the empty center of the being of structures, because he believes the metaphor is "human-sized" (i.e., God is constructed in a human image) and psychologically healthy.

Philosopher Nagel (1986), in his text on objectivity and rationality, takes a different position regarding the empty center: "Some people believe in an afterlife. I do not; what I say will be based on the assumption that death is nothing, and final. I believe there is little to be said for it; it is a great curse, and if we truly face it nothing can make it palatable . . ." (p. 224). Although Nagel is talking about existence after death and Jung about the God metaphor, they are both dealing with the design question about the structure of life and knowing. Nagel makes a judgment on the issue of an afterlife, a position that seems in contrast with his general thesis of the ultimate irresolvability of such fundamental human questions.

We could say that Nagel (1986) has been unable to decenter in his analysis of death. He is egocentrically captured by time's arrow and is completely identified with the ego complex. He then falls prey to the belief that there is but one way to objectify his subjective experience, his feelings about the end of his own individuality. He is unable to consider the question of the meaning of life or death apart from his own individuality.

Jung might contend that Nagel's problem in identifying his experience exclusively with time's arrow, or the ego complex, arises from a psychological state that interferes with the relativizing of the ego (decentering of ego complex) in the second half of life. In *Aion* (CW 9, II), Jung describes two clinical syndromes with similar outcomes: one is the ego's assimilation to the self, and the other is the self's assimilation to the ego. In both, one witnesses an egocentrism that appears as inflated or exaggerated self-importance. Nagel appears to suffer the second type. Jung describes the second type as a psychological inflation of knowing, a "just so" attitude about reality. Neurotic defenses such as reaction formation, intellectualization, sublimation, and humor protect this attitude of "knowing all about" the nature of psyche and even one's own nature. Psychological phenomena such as dreams, metaphors, symbols, and images are then reduced to concrete aspects of brain or physiological behavior that can be understood as "only" this or that. Various forms of realism and positivism can be identified with this kind of egocentrism.

The other type of egocentrism is one in which "the image of wholeness . . . remains in the unconscious, so that on one the hand it shares the archaic nature of the unconscious and on the other finds itself in the psychically relative space–time continuum that is characteristic of the unconscious as such" (CW 9, II, p. 24). This condition appears in borderline and narcissistic personality states, and in various forms of dissociation and altered states of consciousness. People who are convinced of their omniscience, of their ability to see "beyond" or "behind" the ordinary states of time and space, may be understood to suffer from this kind of egocentrism. Their experience of time's arrow is disrupted, and they seem to be living "elsewhere." Although this kind of experience is legitimately a part of religious inspiration, childbirth, shock, grief, and other altered states, it is pathological to live continuously within it. A person possessed by such an archetypal identification with the self may attempt, in fact, to persuade others that she/he is "the" epistemic subject, and hence become the voice that hastens to fill the emptiness of the center, as Broughton worried could happen. Totalitarianism, authoritarianism, and fundamentalism are societal examples of this kind of identification or assimilation of the ego to the self.

JUNG'S ANSWER TO PIAGET

Although Jung characterized the archetypal self as a subject without a subjectivity (as pure form), he seemed intuitively unable to embrace the completely empty center. In this last period of his work, Jung speculated on the nature of the epistemic subject, the "designer" of self design. Whereas Piaget investigated the epistemic subject through studies, especially on children and adolescents, of the development of logical reasoning and empirical thought, Jung investigated individuation through comparative studies of religion and mythology. Jung was especially interested in representations of unity and conflict, and of quest and development.

> Unity and totality stand at the highest point on the scale of objective values because their symbols can no longer be distinguished from the *imago Dei*. Hence all statements about the god-image apply also to the empirical symbols of totality. Experience shows that individual mandalas are symbols of *order*, and that they occur in patients principally during times of psychic disorientation or reorientation. (CW 9, II, pp. 31–32)

What Jung discovered in his investigation of Christ as a symbol of the self (reported in CW 9, II) was that Christ and the Anti-Christ are in an interdependent relationship with each other. Jung believed this was the reason why Jesus is depicted as having been crucified between two thieves: "This great symbol tells us that the progressive development and differentiation of consciousness leads to an ever more menacing awareness of the conflict and involves nothing less than a crucifixion of the ego, its agonizing suspension between two irreconcilable opposites" (CW 9, II, p. 44). Jung came to see these opposites as the dichotomies of human desires and values: love and hate, good and bad, pure and evil, right and wrong. The necessary progress of development is the integration into awareness of the meanings of both sides of the opposites. To say this another way, individuation is an awakening to the suffering within oneself and to one's conflict of desires. An awareness of this struggle in oneself includes an awareness of it in others, and of the irreconcilable difficulties of human life. Such an awakening results in openness to symbolic meaning as well as an appreciation of psychological insight: "anyone who is destined to descend into a deep pit had better set about it with all the necessary precautions rather than risk falling into the hole backwards" (CW 9, II, p. 70).

Jung's study of the Christ image, of medieval philosophy, and of gnosticism, in particular, led him to become interested in the dual nature of divinity. The history of the Western god-image, traced from ancient Hebrew psychology and religion to modern European beliefs about God and Satan, revealed to Jung a *"complexio oppositorum"*—the existence of opposites that may be represented as one god figure, or as a composite split into two or more. Jung became especially interested in the Job story because this depiction of god and man had been perplexing both on religious and psychological grounds. Late in his career, just after Jung had completed *Aion* and his study of the Christ symbolization, he launched into a dialogue with Job.

What resulted was a monograph entitled *The Answer to Job* (CW, 11); few of Jung's writings are so emotionally charged and personally revealing as this one. Jung enters into the story, as it were, in order to discover just what kind of being Yahweh is. In effect, he seeks an answer to the question "What is the subjectivity of the epistemic subject?"—at least for the case of Yahweh. Here is a summary of the portrait he paints:

> The picture of a God who knew no moderation in his emotions and suffered precisely from this lack. . . . Such a condition is only conceivable either when no reflecting consciousness is present at all, or when the capacity for reflection is very feeble and a more or less adventitious phenomenon. A condition of this sort can only be described as *amoral*. (italics in original, CW 11, p. 365)

Jung depicts a god who is in need of man, a god suffering from his lack of conscious discrimination. In essence, Yahweh "forgets" about his omniscience; as Jung says, he fails to consult his omniscience in order to

understand himself or Job. Yahweh is not simply a blending of opposites, according to Jung; rather, he is an "antinomy" or a complete
paradox. This is the "indispensable condition" for his power and knowledge. Unself-reflective and amoral, Yahweh is both envious and awed by
the self-reflection and morality that he witnesses in Job.

Comparing Yahweh to the Greek gods, Jung remarks that Zeus was
far more remote and detached from the human world, largely un-
interested in the affairs of mortals. Zeus only demanded sacrifices, but
he was not interested in the motives of humankind. Yahweh is interested, even attached, to humans: "Human beings were a matter of
first-rate importance to him. He needed them as they needed him,
urgently and personally" (CW 11, p. 370).

So here is Jung's most complete account of the Western epistemic
subject; a perspective that evolves through our own human consciousness, hopelessly emotional and reactive without it. Only to be known as
he is reflected, Yahweh needs "the acclamation of a small group of
people" (CW 11, p. 370). Specifically, Jung says, "Unconsciousness
has an animal nature. Like all old gods Yahweh has his animal symbolism with its unmistakable borrowings from the much older theriomorphic
gods of Egypt . . ." (CW 11, p. 383). Through Job, Yahweh comes to
appreciate that human consciousness is superior to his own in its ability
to reflect on itself. Hence, God is moved to become human, to enter into
this mortal plane of existence in order to experience self-consciousness.
"One should make clear to oneself what it means when God becomes
man. It means nothing less than a world-shaking transformation of God.
It means more or less what Creation meant in the beginning, namely an
objectivation of God" (p. 401). The differentiation of human consciousness, with its peculiar ability to create and sustain a unified self, is a
further development of God, according to Jung. The epistemic subject
becomes conscious of itself through the operations of the human mind.
The epistemic subject has no ability to reflect its own oppositional
nature, or its own contradictory aims. Hence, Yahweh is "morally
defeated" by a "higher" being (Job), and so Yahweh concedes to become
the god–man of Jesus Christ.

At about the same time that the Job story was recorded (some time
between 600 and 300 B.C.E.), Gautama the Buddha (born 562 B.C.E.)
developed a practice of disciplining consciousness as the ultimate goal
of human life. The teachings of the living Buddha explicitly deny the
worship of any god-image. Instead, the practice of conscious discrimination, through compassion for other beings, is elevated over and above the
highest Brahman gods. Conscious discrimination is similarly the goal of
the god called Yahweh. Job's suffering is directly related to the condition
of Yahweh's knowledge prior to his incarnation as a man: concrete and

immediate, embedded in his own being and unable to decenter and reflect on itself. As physicist Freeman Dyson (1988) said, and as we quoted him earlier, "God . . . learns and grows as the universe unfolds" (p. 119). According to Jung, human consciousness is the farthest reach of consciousness in our known universe and the only available moral order.

Dyson (1988) reluctantly admits that he too would make an "argument from design" for a principle of unity between the world and human knowledge. He calls his argument "theological" rather than "scientific," and he says that there is "evidence from peculiar features of the laws of nature that the universe as a whole is hospitable to the growth of mind. . . . Therefore it is reasonable to believe in the existence of . . . a mental component of the universe" (p. 297). Dyson also poses the question of Job: Why do we suffer? His answer is similar to Jung's:

> The universe is constructed according to a principle of maximum diversity. The principle of maximum diversity operates both at the physical and at the mental level. It says that the laws of nature and the initial conditions are such as to make the universe as interesting as possible. (p. 298)

Human self-reflection and our ability to study our own symbolizing processes insure such maximum diversity. To make objective our own subjectivity is to make us capable of discerning our own motives and transcending our limits again and again. This same reflective capacity results in a foreknowledge of our death and a desire to control the related anxiety. Our form of self-reflection leads to the possibility of a morality of choice or free will, but it also leads to the desire to dominate and control. Jung says in his concluding passage on Job: "Everything now depends on man: immense power of destruction is given into his hand, and the question is whether he can resist the will to use it, and can temper his will with the spirit of his own unaided resources" (CW 11, 459).

SYNCHRONICITY AND THE SPACE-MIND OF SELF

Jung's well-known essay "Synchronicity: An Acausal Connecting Principle" was published first in 1952, although many of its major tenets were laid down in Jung's (CW 11) commentaries on Eastern religions and Western gnosticism. Like other readers, we have been impressed by the compelling nature of his arguments, but troubled by the lack of explanatory concepts and the generally weak experimental evidence. Yet we have found the concept of synchronicity useful. Like other therapists we have found ourselves with inadequate explanations for the rare occasions of discovering the "day residue" meaning of a dream in the day *after*, rather than the day before the dream. These kinds of "coincidences" violate our usual understanding of time's arrow and seem to require some other theory of time or causality. Jung's idea of synchronicity as an "acausal connecting principle" has had appeal for many psychologists and scientists. His definition of it from the essay is as follows:

> Synchronicity . . . means the simultaneous occurrence of a certain psychic state with one or more external events which appear as meaningful parallels to the momentary subjective state—and, in certain cases, vice versa. (CW 8, p. 441)

Examples of these occurrences given by Jung include such events as parapsychological experiments in which motivated subjects are able to choose correctly from a group of stimuli presented to them (e.g., a deck of cards) the corresponding images or themes represented by the experimenter or others who are outside of the normal reaches of space and time in the subjects' perception. These subjects demonstrate abilities and skills that are similar to the dream's depiction of the day-after meaning. Such situations violate our experience of time's arrow and the usual limitations of human knowledge. People appear to "know" things they cannot know, given our typical understanding of space, time, and causality. Other examples given by Jung include the "chance" presentation of animals and numbers in the environment just at the moment when they are emotionally significant (e.g., appearing also in a dream or personal fantasy). Jung stresses that these kinds of events include both objective data of sense perceptions *and* subjective experience of emotional significance.

Synchronous events are always emotionally motivated from the point of view of the subject, and this motivation has to be distinguished from wishing and "magical thinking," which connects momentary intersubjective reality with one's psychological complexes (more about that later). Jung also differentiates synchronous events from mere chance events that have no particular emotional significance (e.g., two friends buying the same shoes).

Jung is, to some extent, always arguing "against" or in opposition to a purely causal model for psychology. Many theorists (e.g., systems, cybernetics, and hermeneutic theorists) now reject a purely causal model for psychology on grounds different from Jung's. We can discern in Jung's discussion a constructivist meaning that is uniquely useful. The connection of perceptual facts of experience (including time, space, and causality) with *personal meaning* is the revolutionary contribution Jung makes in his theory of synchronicity.

Jung focuses especially on "affectivity" involved in synchronous events. He recalls the fact that parapsychological experiments tend to fail as soon as the subjects become bored, distracted, or otherwise no longer motivated to succeed. As we have discussed archetypes in this and other chapters, it is apparent that emotional arousal is the essential component for the coherence and experience of archetypes in everyday life. Archetypal dreams, for example, are highly charged emotional events. Such dreams, Jung suggests, may be uniquely motivating during times of resistance and standstill in analysis:

> If they are serious enough, archetypal dreams are likely to occur which point out a possible line of advance one would never have thought of oneself. It is this kind of situation that constellates the archetype with the greatest regularity. In certain cases the psychotherapist therefore sees himself obliged to discover the rationally insoluble problem towards which the patient's unconscious is steering. (CW 8, pp. 440–441)

Jung's point here is that a standstill in the therapeutic process may produce dream material that advances the therapeutic work without the anticipation of the client or therapist. It is precisely the affective charge of the moment, from Jung's perspective, that provides the ground for such a synchronous experience.

Jung, like many physicists, believes that "space and time . . . are probably at bottom one and the same" (CW 8, p. 445), but there is a paucity of explanatory power in his statements such as the following:

> Synchronistic events rest on the *simultaneous occurrence of two different psychic states*. One of them is the normal, probable state (i.e., the one that is causally explicable), and the other, the critical experience, is the one that cannot be derived causally from the first. (italics in original, pp. 444–445)

Jung has difficulty transcending Kant—reasoning outside of the categories of space, time, and causality. That is, although Jung attempts to extend Kantian categories, he is usually bound to Kantian explanations for categories of mind or knowledge. For example, he says in *Aion* in 1950, "The space–time quaternio is the archetypal *sine qua non* for any apprehension of the physical world—indeed, the very possibility of apprehending it. It is the organizing schema par excellence among the psychic quaternities" (CW 9, II, p. 253).

As we have already stressed, we believe that archetypal theory is better explained within the context of *embodiment theory* than within Kantian mentalism. Human embodiment can thus be taken as the organizing form, constraint, and boundary for human mental categories, as well as the origin of image-schemata of space, time, and causality. The invariants of human subjectivity (agency, coherence, continuity, and emotional arousal) are the principles for our consensual construction of reality, in both its physical and mental properties. As many philosophers and psychologists have now recognized, human agency appears to be our model for causality. Similarly, coherence or unity of body-being is the foundation for our experiences of point of view and space (both space "within" and "outside" the body). Continuity is the basis of time organization. And, finally, emotional arousal can impinge on or disrupt any of the others, *and* provides apparently the situational factors for image-thinking.

Jung is concerned to show that statistical methods and causality are limited paradigms for psychology. He wants to stress the importance of the psychological "moment" in the capacity to organize images, but he finds it difficult to break with the Kantian model. In effect, Jung decides to add "synchronicity" as another Kantian category. Jung is aware of the development of relativism and observer phenomena in physics (e.g., "causality is bound up with the existence of space and time and physical changes, and consists essentially in the succession of cause and effect" (CW 8, pp. 445–446), but he is unable to assimilate this kind of relativism to psychological theory per se. We believe that we are now able to do this.

The influences of constructivism and contemporary critical disciplines, and to a lesser extent the assimilation of Buddhist philosophy to occidental beliefs, permit us to develop a new psychological understanding of the principle of synchronicity. The effects of the *moment* of emotional arousal on the psychological construction of images are better apprehended now than in the 1950s when Jung was trying to articulate his theory. For example, Guidano and Liotti (1983) write:

> Every human being from the very beginning actively processes two flows of stimuli that, through belonging to different levels, are always simultaneous: perception of the world and self-perception. Thus, any information about the outside world always and inevitably corresponds to information about self. In this way the elaboration of knowledge appears to be a unitary process that occurs through a dynamic interplay of two polarities, the self and world, which can be metaphorically equated to the two sides of a coin: a subject's self-knowledge always involves his or her conception of reality, and . . . conversely, every conception of reality is directly connected to the subject's view of self. (p. 108)

These theorists go on to stress the role of attachment in establishing the "reality" of the world. Emotional arousal in attachment relationships, in experiences of bonding and separation, establishes the basis for reality perception.

Although Jung's ideas do not focus on bonding or the relational underpinnings of image-formation, they contain the seeds for understanding the essentially interpersonal nature of reality construction. The relational domain, as the central link between self-knowledge and knowledge of the world, is the arena of emotional arousal and archetypal experiences. Assuming that human knowledge is structured through the affective particulars of both early and later attachment relationships (i.e., attachments to caregivers and to adult partners), we argue that synchronicity is related primarily to the consensual validation of affective meaning in an aroused state. The validation of an image as affectively meaningful—related both to the subject's arousal and existing as a momentary phenomenon—typically takes place in a relational context. Usually the relationship is between two people—for instance, the "recipient" and the "sender" of psychic messages or the recognition by the therapist that the client's bizarre experiences were "real." A more abstract relationship, as between a book (such as the Chinese oracle, *The I Ching*) and a person, is potentially one of affective validation but is more problematic. The "recipient" of the synchronistic message, in this case, cannot easily validate the affective meaning except in reference to subjective experience. Mere projection of subjective meaning onto the phenomenal world is more easily checked within an interpersonal relationship than within an intrapsychic one. Because synchronistic events specifically violate our usual experiences of agency (causality), coherence (space), and continuity (time), they are necessarily rare and disruptive.

If a person experiences such disruptive events frequently, there is a problem in the continuity and coherence of self, as we mentioned above—and usually the problem is one of psychotic disruption, traumatic loss or abuse, or severe illness. These latter experiences are acute or painful ones in which the typical dimensions of consensual reality are disrupted. Synchronistic events are not psychotic events. Because synchronistic events form a "special case" or an exception to the rule of consensual validation, they specifically illustrate the ongoing consensual nature of reality construction.

Self and world are constructed in the emotionally charged states of early and later attachment relationships. When all goes well, the affective particulars of psychological complexes are matched closely enough between and among individuals, that people agree on a typical phenomenal world rooted in the invariants of subjectivity. When we do not privilege the physical world as a "source" of phenomenal reality, then we see that synchronicity emerges as a special case that makes apparent the usual psychological nature of meaning construction. Synchronous events are the rare occasions in which *individual* emotional arousal serves as a structuring principle for an event in the phenomenal world that can be validated by another person or knowledge system as meaningful. The affective particulars of the meaning system are agreed on by the people participating in the emotional moment who validate it as a synchronous event.

As we discuss in more detail later, the central propositions of both the original teachings of Buddhist philosophy and later teachings of Mahayana Buddhism fit nicely into a constructivist model of subjectivity and can support a theory of synchronicity. In a brief discussion of principles of Mahayana Buddhism, Blofeld (1977) talks about the cognitive nature of phenomenal reality and its basis in a shared mentality:

> It is taught that reality has two aspects—the realms of Void and form—but that, due to obscurations arising from primordial ignorance, . . . we fail to *see* that nothing can exist independently of everything else, that all entities (including people) are transient, mutable, unsatisfying and *lacking in own-being*. . . . The way out lies within each sentient being's mind in the form of latent wisdom—compassion. . . . This is so because so-called individual minds are not truly apart from Mind, the Plenum in which everything exists forever and forever. (p. 88)

Western psychologies usually assume that mind is individual and separate, rather than shared and expansive (in which "everything" exists "forever and forever"). In this and other chapters, we have encountered Piaget's concept of epistemic subject, Jung's model of individuation, and our own (and others') invariants of subjectivity, all of which are versions of universal mind or the principle of developing structure in the universe. Jung's theory of synchronicity is an attempt to allow for exceptional and explicit demonstrations of universal mind when they occur in human experiences. It is an effort to make the theory of universal mind an empirically testable hypothesis that can be demonstrated according to certain rules of validation.

Blofeld (1977) presents the idea of universal mind in another way also. He gives accounts of certain of the great masters of advanced abstract practices of Buddhism (such as Ch'an or Zen) showing that these masters refuse to invalidate the "reality" of animism and similar beliefs in "concrete" appearances of Buddhas and the like.

> Even exceedingly erudite Buddhists . . . hold that the various Pure
> Lands . . . do in a sense exist as places, since mind has thus
> conceived them. This seemingly startling departure from logic is
> somewhat less puzzling if one accepts that *all* entities are mental
> creations, none ultimately more or less real than any other. (1977,
> p. 89)

Synchronistic occurrences can thus be explained as mental creations
that are meaningful for people who are emotionally involved with practices or events that are known to produce such images.

Jung's most frequent examples of synchronous events are those
involving traumatic or peak emotional experiences, such as the death of
a close relative or the tense standstill of therapeutic process. In such
moments, the phenomenal world may "re-present" aspects of psychic
meaning for the people who are so aroused. For example, a clock stops at
the time of its owner's death, or a distant relative (unaware of an
imminent death) dreams of the death. Similarly a highly motivated
subject of an experiment may be able to perceive the "re-presentation"
of certain stimuli held in the mind of another person. People sharing
these kinds of experiences usually state that they feel unable to "prove"
to others that their explanations are meaningful because they cannot
invoke usual rational and causal categories.

Jung believed that Western psychology would be hard put to come
to terms with the "impersonal Universal Mind" of Buddhism. "In the
East, the mind is a cosmic factor, the very essence of existence; while in
the West we have just begun to understand that it is the essential
condition of cognition, and hence of the cognitive existence of the world"
(CW 11, p. 480). And yet even this statement indicates that cognitive
psychology—and now its formalization in constructivism—might someday be receptive to the principal tenets of a theory of universal mind.

STRUCTURE AND DYNAMICS OF SELF

> In the end we have to acknowledge that the self is a *complexio*
> *oppositorum* precisely because there can be no reality without polar-
> ity. We must not overlook the fact that opposites acquire their moral
> accentuation only within the sphere of human endeavour and action,
> and that we are unable to give a definition of good and evil that could
> be considered universally valid. (CW 9, II, p. 267)

Jung undertook to write a volume explicitly about the self because
he had received repeated requests to relate the "natural symbols" of

wholeness—such as mandalas, religious stories of exemplary lives, and images of central value (such as sun, atom, etc.)—to the cultural image of Jesus Christ. Connecting the Christ-symbol with the Anthropos (the "Son of Man") and associating it with the development of spiritual consciousness in human embodiment, Jung sought to provide a psychological analysis of the development of symbolic forms through the particular development of Christianity, Gnosticism, and alchemy. The structure of *Aion* (CW 9, II) is divided between topics of Jungian theory associated with the self—such as ego, shadow, and anima/animus—and topics of Christianity, Gnosticism, and alchemy. In two chapters, for example, Jung discusses fish symbolism as it is associated with Christianity and alchemy, emphasizing especially the *ambivalence* of the fish that represents both good and bad, in that it is both sustaining and devouring. In the penultimate chapter, he presents his theory of the structure and dynamics of self as a universal model of individuation.

Jung employs the motif of a traditional cross-cousin marriage to introduce the central notion of tension or opposition within subjectivity. The cross-cousin marriage pattern, from anthropological studies, requires that a man marry his mother's brother's daughter, and that a woman marry her father's sister's son. The line of appropriate connection for further development of an individual is, then, passed through the parent of the opposite sex to the cousin of the opposite sex. This sets up a kind of tension between endogamous attachments to the family and the exogamous connections to the world or tribe. People are required to move away from the family of origin, at some distance, but also to remain within the boundaries of the family's interest.

Jung uses this motif of cross-cousin marriage to describe the intrapsychic dynamics of the relationship of the ego complex to the anima or animus complex (depending on the gender of the person). The ego assimilates psychological experience to itself with the force of endogamous libido. That is, individual subjectivity has a primary interest in itself, argues Jung, in a manner similar to Nagel (1986), who says,

> The internal awareness of my own existence carries with it a particularly strong sense of its own future, and of its possible continuation beyond any future that may actually be reached. It is stronger than the sense of future possibility attaching to the existence of any particular thing in the world objectively conceived—perhaps of a strength surpassed only by the sense of possible continuation we have about the world itself. (p. 226)

For Jung, however, this function of attachment to individual subjectivity is counterbalanced by another psychological complex, representing the exogamous dynamic of connection to the world. The anima complex (of male femininity) in the man, or the animus complex (of female masculinity) in the woman, is the psychological organization of this exogamous connection. After reaching sexual maturity, the projection of the anima or animus onto a person of the opposite sex may bind the ego to the otherness (of world and unconscious) and hence provide the tension for individuation. The contrasexual complex may also be projected onto aspects of the external environment (e.g., science or religion) that come to be desired and/or known through love. From Jung's point of view, the tension between endogamous and exogamous desires is "given" in the nature of subjectivity, especially in maturity when it is experienced as unresolvable conflict.

In the mature adult, there is then a tension between ego and world that contrasts with the experience of unity that is the archetypal self. In *Aion*, Jung defines the archetypal self as "the archetype that underlies ego-consciousness" (p. 222). We argue that the evidence for this archetype appears both in the ubiquitous form of the human body and in the invariants of subjectivity. Jung argues that the evidence is given in images and symbols of wholeness—in people's dreams, creative expressions, and cultural rituals.

> The most important of these [symbols of the self] are geometrical structures containing elements of the circle and quaternity. . . . quadratic figures divided into four or in the form of a cross. They can also be four objects or persons related to one another in meaning or by the way they are arranged . . . From here the analogy formation leads on to the city, castle, church, house, room, and vessel. Another variant is the wheel. (CW 9, II, pp. 223–224)

Especially the house, room, and vessel emphasize "the ego's containment in the greater dimension of the self," and the wheel illustrates "the rotation which also appears as a ritual circumambulation" (p. 224). Jung fails to note here, that embodiment itself might suggest the container and contained motifs, as Johnson (1987) has fully demonstrated.

Jung's description of the self in this volume forms a parallel with his description of Yahweh in *The Answer to Job*, and hence we could assume that he considers *Aion* to be a further exploration of the epistemic subject. The self, like Yahweh, is described as "paradoxical, antinomial. . . . male and female, old man and child, powerful and helpless, large and small. . . . a true *complexio oppositorum*, though this does not mean that it is anything like as contradictory in itself" (italics in original, CW 9, II, p. 225). The contradictions, Jung supposes, may appear to us only through our observing the changes in conscious attitude (from one position to its opposite) rather than actual contradictions in the self. Between conscious and unconscious, Jung asserts that "there is a kind of *uncertainty relationship* because the observer is inseparable from the observed and always disturbs it by the act of observation of the conscious and vice versa" (italics in original, CW 9 II, p. 226).

Jung presents a series of diagrams that depict what he takes to be the archetypal form of the self, and he places them into a dynamic continuum that portrays a spiral developmental process. The images and models used by Jung to depict individuation are associated primarily with Gnosticism, alchemy, and the Old Testament. Most contemporary psychologists and psychotherapists have little knowledge of these topics and would benefit little from learning the names attached to the diagrams. Consequently, we summarize the meaning of the diagrams and present some examples, using generic terms (such as "sister" or "father").

First Jung offers a model of the psychological tension of endogamous and exogamous desires. Figure 5.1 is an illustration of this model from the perspective of the male personality (the perspective presented by Jung).

Husband————————————————————Cousin as Wife
Husband's Sister————————————————Wife's Brother

FIGURE 5.1

Jung claims that the cross-cousin marriage motif represents a "great cultural advance" over the sister-exchange marriage, the older "biological character" of marriage. In the sister-exchange marriage, the sister's husband is the wife's brother, but in the cross-cousin motif the husband is a more distant relative or even a stranger. Jung assumes that the alchemical representation of the "marriage quaternio" (in the form of the cross-cousin marriage motif) is an indication of the psychological development of marriage, and by extension of the self, in the mature personality. Now that the husband and wife are more distant relatives (or strangers) they take on "exalted rank" and "magical powers" that point to contrasexual projection. As Jung says, "marriage has become *psychologically* complicated. It is no longer a state of mere biological and social coexistence, but is beginning to turn into a conscious relationship" (CW 9, II, pp. 242–243). Because of the increasing strangeness of the marriage partner, connection occurs through psychological projection of unconscious complexes (i.e., the anima or animus) rather than through the familiarity of immediate family attachment.

Jung claims that this model of psychological development has both a favorable and an unfavorable aspect. The favorable one is represented in Fig. 5.1 as a conscious relationship, but the unfavorable one is represented as an "incestuous" relationship that depicts unconscious meanings. In the unfavorable arrangement, the husband is represented as the Father (in-law) who is married to the Mother–Sister–Anima. This combination produces a Daughter–Sister–Anima who is married to the mother's brother. In this kind of unconscious relationship there is a chaotic connection of endogamous themes rather than a conscious connection of exogamous meaning (Fig. 5.2).

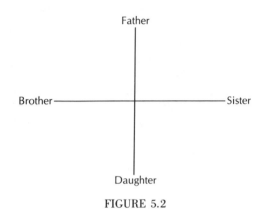

FIGURE 5.2

This incestuous (endogamous) pattern is the complement to the ordered (exogamous) pattern of conscious relationships. It is immaterial whether we understand the particular dynamics Jung is attempting to relate. We need understand only that the marriage quaternio represents *both* the endogamous pull of intrapsychic assimilation (symbolically incestuous or unconscious dynamics), *and* the exogamous pull of extrapsychic accommodation (conscious differentiation through the relationship). The desire to move "forward" or to become conscious is what Jung calls a "dilemma" psychologically. As he states it, one must move beyond both the two- and three-person relationships of early family life into a fourth position of "order" or culture. The fourth position allows one to see the meaning of the entire design.

Jung believes that the Father image (represented by the Husband and Father in the above models), in men, is the image-schematum of "guide" or mentor of development of the archetypal self during the mature years. The Sister–Anima is a more ambivalent figure because this complex can link a man to the incestuous motif of Mother–Sister endogamous meaning *or* to the Wife–World exogamous meaning.

The various points of view from which Jung describes the model of the cross-cousin marriage illustrate the psychological experience of the ego having a "portable identity" as a relatively fixed set of images that fluctuate within personal identity. Individual subjectivity may be experienced as gendered self, as Father complex, as Sister–Anima, or as Mother–Daughter. Thus, the developing *male* ego complex has several perspectives from which to create meaning. Jung is attempting to fill out a structure for subjectivity that is grounded in culture and mediated by the psychological images that arise in the unconscious to constitute the world. Another set of images comprises the *female* ego complex (see Young-Eisendrath & Wiedemann, 1987), but with the same underlying logic of opposing pulls and incestuous themes. Identity images of the self may be projected and experienced as being "out there," or identified as individual subjectivity "in here."

In *The Book of the Self* (Young-Eisendrath & Hall, 1987), we rendered a similar model to illustrate the development of self from the state of personal being. Figure 5.3 represents our attempt to depict a developmental process without the specific grounding in the cultural forms used by Jung. Our model is an adaptation of Harré's (1984) schema to illustrate the development of individual subjectivity. Our

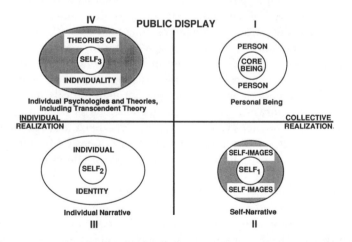

FIGURE 5.3. From *The Book of the Self: Person, Pretext, Process* (p. 455) by P. Young-Eisendrath and J. Hall, 1987, New York: New York University Press. Copyright 1987 by New York University Press. Reprinted by permission.

first quadrant represents the public and collective construct of *person*. The core being state of the person is organized by the invariants of subjectivity—the archetype of self. Typically, all people develop individual subjectivity as point of view and point of action. This experience is captured and recorded in self-images organized into a continuous narrative, recorded in semantic and episodic memory after the emergence of self-conscious emotions (e.g., pride, shame, guilt, envy). Our Self 1 in Figure 5.3 is equivalent to Jung's model of the cross-cousin marriage. Jung fills out his model with particular images from alchemy and Christianity. We simply note that self-images are formed (or "talked into being") around gender, social roles, and the like, within the family of origin and initial social groups. In our model, we assume that the self develops within a culture of persons who consider themselves to be psychological individuals. This experience, mapped onto quadrant III, is assumed to take place differently depending on how a culture fosters individuality. The final quadrant in our model depicts a domain of self-reflexive discourse in which people (psychological individuals) engender various models of individual subjectivity—Jung's model being one of these. Whereas we had in mind merely a mapping of the individuation process relative to cultural context, Jung had in mind a *universal* mapping of an "unfolding of the unknowable inchoate state, or chaos" (CW 9, II, p. 237) into the multiplicity of phenomenal forms in human consciousness.

Jung assumes that the quaternity form is itself an "organizing schema par excellence" and "a system of coordinates that is used almost instinctively for dividing up and arranging a chaotic multiplicity" (CW 9, II, p. 242). He cites the many ways in which we ordinarily sort into four parts, such as seasons, directions, colors, phases of the moon, etc. But he also asserts that clinical evidence shows that in creative imaginative productions and in chaotic psychological states (such as loss and psychosis), quaternity symbols appear and "signify stabilization through order as opposed to the instability caused by chaos" (p. 243).

Jung uses the quaternity to illustrate a progressive spiral development of human consciousness in a model of genetic epistemology that is both phylogenetic and ontogenetic. He uses the figure developed by the idea of cross-cousin marriage to illustrate a tension of opposites at progressive levels of differentiation of the self–world. Vertically the figure looks like the following (Fig. 5.4), in which each level of dynamic tension (expressed as a diamond shape) represents a particular level of differentiation. Each level is a reorganization of all the others; the levels move from chaos, to mineral, to animal, to human, and finally to "anthropos" or divinized human. Each level is represented in tension with every other but is organized as parts within an identical whole.

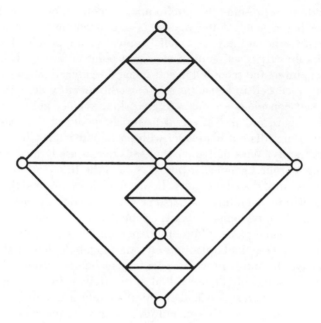

FIGURE 5.4. Jung's hierarchical self. From *The Collected Works of C. G. Jung: Aion* (p. 247) by C. G. Jung, 1959, Princeton, NJ: Princeton University Press. Copyright 1959. Adapted by permission.

As in Blofeld's (1977) account of the universal mind, each level of Jung's model presents an image that is *both* psychological and phenomenological in its organization of consciousness. Thus, the level of animal life (serpent, in Jung's language) is meant to encompass both the phenomenon of animal life and animal consciousness *and* the symbolic meaning of "animal" consciousness in human experience. Each level is thus both experience and analog, as the process unfolds. Ultimately Jung arranges this model to create a mandala in which his genetic epistemology takes on a "spiral" character, imagined to be moving "forward" as with time's arrow, and a "mandala" character, imagined to be stable as with time's cycle. The final figure is seen in Figure 5.5.

With the help of these models, Jung discusses the organization of the physical world of time, space, and energy according to its "psychoid" nature, or the way in which it appears to interact with human mentation—the idea of a universe hospitable to mental development.

The complete formula presented by Jung is a model of transformation and integration, depicted as "an unfolding of totality into four parts four times, which means nothing less than its becoming conscious" (CW 9, II, p. 259). Jung's rather elaborate development of this metaphor,

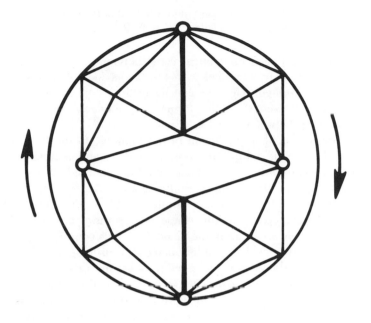

FIGURE 5.5. Jung's transformative self. From *The Collected Works of C. G. Jung: Aion* (p. 248) by C. G. Jung, 1959, Princeton, NJ: Princeton University Press. Copyright 1959. Adapted by permission.

primarily from alchemical sources, is his effort to set forth an image of a psychological universe at the interface between knower and known.

> The formula presents a symbol of the self, for the self is not just a static quantity or constant form, but is also a dynamic process. In the same way, the ancients saw the *imago Dei* in man not as a mere imprint . . . but as an active force. The four transformations represent a process of restoration or rejuvenation taking place, as it were, inside the self, and comparable to the carbon–nitrogen cycle in the sun. . . . The carbon nucleus itself comes out of the reaction unchanged . . . The secret of existence, i.e., the existence of the atom and its components, may well consist in a continually repeated process of rejuvenation. . . . (CW 9, II, p. 260)

Jung acknowledges the "extremely hypothetical nature" of his comparison between the sun's cycle and the self, but then goes on to make a constructivist argument in favor of his position.

> Since analogy formation is a law which to a large extent governs the life of the psyche, we may fairly conjecture that our—to all appear-

ances—purely speculative construction is not a new invention, but is
prefigured on earlier levels of thought. (CW 9, II, p. 261)

Jung observes here that mathematical constructions that "transcend all
experience" have often coincided with the "behaviour of things" after
they have been invented. Thus we can have direct knowledge that our
forms of thought intersect with other forms in the universe, expressing an
ultimate harmony between forms of existence.

Jung returns, in the conclusion of the chapter, to the basic con-
stituents of the self, in its differentiation: shadow, anima/animus, and
the *complexio oppositorum*. Psychologically, Jung contends that conflict
or the union of opposites is the essential notion. Abstractly, the self
stands for "psychic totality," Jung reiterates, but "Empirically . . . the
self appears spontaneously in the shape of specific symbols, and its
totality is discernible above all in the mandala and its countless variants.
Historically, these symbols are authenticated as God-images" (CW 9, II,
p. 268). In the development of religion, Jung assumes that the animus/
anima stage of ambivalent desires (described above) depicts "polythe-
ism" and that the recognition of the unity of the self is expressed in
"monotheism." The most fruitful attempts to express symbols of the self,
in Jung's view, are set forth by the alchemists and the Gnostics. They
were especially successful because they "allowed themselves to be
influenced in large measure by natural inner experience" (p. 269).

In Evelyn Fox Keller's (1985) revealing essay on "Spirit and Reason
at the Birth of Modern Science," the author presents an elaborate
analysis of the interaction between early modern scientists and alchemists in the 17th century. She makes the argument that alchemy was
rejected primarily because of its investment in the full nature of experience. She says that for alchemists "God was immanent in the material
world, in woman, and in sexuality" and for the rational scientists,
"chastity was a condition for Godliness; and truth . . . was the province
of the dispassionate intellect" (p. 59). The point that she ultimately
makes is that modern science has inexorably separated knowledge and
desire, the knower and the known.

Alchemy, by contrast, emphasized "illumination derived from direct experience (available to anyone who pursues the art)," and its tenets
(especially those established in the works of Paracelsus) "captured the
imagination of many thinkers, including the members of the Oxford
Group (a precursor of the Royal Society) but were perhaps especially
attractive to political and religious radicals" (pp. 45–46). In the final
analysis, states Keller, the alchemists were threatening to the mechani-
cal scientists not only because of their methods and their radicalism but,
also, because of their "commitment to a science steeped in erotic sexual

imagery and simultaneously, to the symbolic equality of women before God." Drawing on alchemy for his model of the self, Jung grounded himself in the affective-imaginal experience of symbolic thinking. His biases in theorizing from experience leave us with both strengths and weaknesses in terms of contemporary constructivism. The strengths include the study of direct experience (relative to gender and contra-sexuality especially). Weaknesses involve the conflations of experiences of subjectivity with the design of individuation, a point to be developed further in the last chapter.

This chapter has presented a way of integrating the most radical ideas of Jung's self psychology with the influences of constructivism and other contemporary epistemologies in order to examine the possibilities of relating Jung's ideas to contemporary theories of self.

In the next chapter we present a fragment of a clinical case. The case report involves a middle-aged man who is part-way through a Jungian analysis with Dr. Hall. The analysand is grappling with his parental complexes at a time in his life when he wishes he were more settled and content. We will use the case in the following chapters as a vehicle to illustrate (1) the importance of understanding the self in approaching psychotherapy; (2) the comparative significance of twelve self theories; and (3) finally, the application of Jung's self theory to psychotherapeutic work.

☆6☆

The Self in
Mid-Life: A Case
for Interpretation

The case description that follows is a brief study of a man in his late 40s. He has entered Jungian psychotherapy because of recent losses and doubts about his career development. (His therapy is ongoing at the time of this writing.) Different from many of Jung's own patients who achieved a great deal by midlife, this man has not yet "found himself" in the area of career or family life. Although he was once married, "Jerry" does not look back on the marriage as a fully achieved one. Rather, he now holds out the hope that he might "someday" be able to have a complete relationship with a partner. Similarly, he hopes for a career possibility that will allow him to fulfill himself.

In Jungian terminology, Jerry fits the description of a "puer eternus" or the "eternal youth." This is not quite the same thing as a "narcissistic personality" or the "Peter Pan syndrome," but it is similar. We will discuss this aspect of Jerry's personality when we present the Jungian interpretation of this case in Chapter 8.

In Chapter 7, we present interpretations and theoretical understandings of the case from other points of view. Using a variety of self theories, we attempt to show how the case might be seen in terms of aspects of subjectivity that show through different lenses.

This chapter simply presents the case from Dr. Hall's description of it, leaving out (as much as possible) both theoretical implications and specific interventions. Consider Jerry to be a therapeutic case example to be studied from a number of perspectives.

INTRODUCING JERRY

When Jerry, a 47-year-old man, entered Jungian analysis, he had been divorced for more than 10 years from the mother of his two late-adolescent daughters. The marriage had been largely placid but un-fulfilling for both partners. After the divorce, Jerry and his ex-wife continued on superficially polite and friendly terms, except for disagreements over Jerry's financial contributions to the children's care, particularly when the girls entered college. Jerry took pride in his record of meticulous payment of child support, even during the brief times when he was unemployed. The younger of his two daughters resented that he had not given her more financial help during college, and her feelings were a source of disappointment to him. But he also felt that his not overindulging her, or feeling guilty for saying no, was a part of his fathering and facilitated the development of her independence.

In spite of his disappointment at the failure of his marriage, and the continuing failures of intimate relationships with other women, Jerry believed that he wanted to remarry and to continue family life.

At the initial interview, Jerry looked at least 10 years younger than his stated age. He was trim in weight, and his hair appeared to be styled and neatly in place. He dressed casually in slacks and a shirt that was open several buttons down. His appearance was neat and low key. He chose a chair near the therapist in preference to the couch or a lounge chair with an ottoman. Jerry leaned forward and was animated and emotionally expressive as he told his story. He would frequently take on a pained look, as if reflecting on an inner sense of discomfort. Broadly articulate and obviously well educated, he expressed himself clearly and directly but with frequent references to his uncertainty. He sometimes inquired if the analyst understood him and was "really listening." He would sometimes slouch in the chair with a defeated look, seeming at those times even younger.

In subsequent sessions, he often dressed even more casually, sometimes in jeans with tennis shoes over bare feet. On the rare occasions when he appeared in a suit and tie, it was in preparation for making business presentations to clients later the same day. Although he worked at home alone, with occasional temporary help, he liked to create the impression of a larger office by using a corporate name with the word "associates" in it and having his answering service respond to phone calls as though he had an office with secretaries.

Jerry's motivation for entering psychotherapy at this time was due to persistent fears of inadequacy. He had doubts about his ability to support himself doing consultant work, but at the same time, he did not like the thought of returning to work for a large corporation, which he felt made him vulnerable to sudden dismissal. He was also troubled by recurrent homosexual fantasies that contributed to a problem in making eye contact with men. He dated regularly, however, and had satisfactory heterosexual relationships, but since his divorce he had found it difficult to maintain an intimate relationship with a woman. His masturbation fantasies were heterosexual, often recreating in fantasy sexual experiences with actual women in his past. Though he had sex with women, he had difficulty with delayed ejaculation.

Jerry chose a Jungian analyst (James Hall) because he had had a "strong" reaction to him (in hearing him at a public lecture), which he felt would facilitate his psychotherapy. Although he had experienced this reaction as "not entirely positive," at the conclusion of the initial interview, Jerry was careful to tell Dr. Hall that he liked him and thought that they could work together.

The initial therapeutic contract was for once-a-week individual sessions of 45 minutes, with the possibility of adding group psychotherapy later. He agreed to the regular fee without negotiation, remarking that it was somewhat of a financial struggle, but he thought psychotherapy "was worth it." (Classical Jungian analysis, focusing principally on symbolic material such as dreams, is often done once weekly. Other forms of Jungian analysis, emphasizing the transferential field more, may require more frequent meetings.) Jerry agreed to remember and record his dreams so that dream analysis could be a regular aspect of his treatment.

Jerry's previous experience of psychotherapy had been several years before in an adjacent state. There he had worked with two male psychiatrists who were loosely associated in the same practice. With Dr. B., his major therapist, Jerry had developed a strong relationship. Dr. B. had been both supportive and structuring, often giving what Jerry considered to be good practical advice and insight. He saw the second psychiatrist, Dr. C, at an earlier time when Dr. B. was leading his group psychotherapy. Dr. C. was perceived as less supportive, gave less direction and encouragement, and seemed less important in Jerry's memory.

The possibility of concurrent group psychotherapy had been initially discussed, but a decision was postponed until individual therapy was securely under way, as judged by the establishment of a therapeutic alliance. Group psychotherapy, sometimes an adjunct to Jungian analysis, was suggested in this case in order to afford greater opportunities for emotional interactions (in the group) that would parallel past relational dynamics, current relationships, dreams, and the transference. In

Jerry's case particularly, Dr. Hall believed group therapy would increase the affective experience of interpretation. Jerry had had previous group psychotherapy and had some apprehension about speaking of his problems, particularly his sexual thoughts, in a group of "strangers." Eventually he entered concurrent group psychotherapy and has continued for the last 5 years in both individual and group therapy. (Two sessions of 3 hours each of group psychotherapy per month are accompanied by four once-a-week individual therapy sessions in this model.)

Initially Jerry seemed to present a picture of chronic low-grade "characterological" depression. There was no suicidal ideation or history of suicide attempts. A certain dependent and slightly overly polite tone to Jerry's self-presentation suggested the presence of underlying hostility or anger, a surmise that proved correct within a very few meetings. The precipitating stress for entrance into therapy included losses both in his relational and his work life. As mentioned earlier, Jerry had lost a 6-month relationship with a woman whom he had liked a lot. He had been very attracted to her beauty and apparent competence. She initially seemed warm and accepting, but this dissipated with time, and the relationship became dominated by mutual criticism. Almost simultaneously he lost his job with a large and successful "frontier" company in the computing field. The president of the company (that had rapidly risen to prominence) was a woman, Cynthia. Jerry described her as "having balls." She was very active, extroverted, and creative. Although he claimed that he felt no personal animosity towards her (his being fired was for corporate reasons), he envied her independence and financial success.

His closest friend in the corporation was a woman, Jane, who lost her position at the firm at the same time he did. Although Jerry had had sexual fantasies about her, they had never "officially" been lovers, even though, on some business trips they had shared a room overnight. He continued his friendship with Jane after they had both left the corporation and set up independent and successful consultant businesses for themselves.

Jerry appeared to be a good candidate for Jungian analysis because of his verbal skills and his apparent ability to self-reflect, accompanied by good adaptation and an ability to appreciate metaphorical meaning, such as that depicted in dream images. Jerry seemed capable of controlling his impulses and appreciating personal symbols. To be a good candidate for analysis, one must be able readily to make use of symbolic representation of emotional meanings with minimal risk for acting out within or outside of the transference. Jerry's underlying hostility soon emerged as acting out in the transference, however. He would at times interrupt his narrative with pressured remarks like "I want to hit you!" or

"I want to kick you!" These remarks were always followed by an immediate apologetic statement, and his saying that he was reporting them because they had "simply come to mind" and that he would never, of course, act on any such impulse.

FAMILY OF ORIGIN AND BACKGROUND

Jerry was the younger of two children. His sister Susan was 4 years his senior. Their father "wasn't there" emotionally, preferring to spend leisure time in his woodworking shop in the basement, in the few hours he was home with the family. In childhood Jerry resented his father and even now felt that his father had not been involved sufficiently in his life. It seemed that his father would only interact with the family on the father's own terms, such as long Sunday drives in the mountains. From Jerry's point of view, his father had no awareness of Jerry's interests or desires.

His mother was a strict disciplinarian. She sometimes had made him pull down his pants and spanked his legs with a rubber hose, which she claimed was safer than a switch. Mother also frequently gave enemas (which he hated) as remedies. Sometimes she would speak in her language of origin (not English) with her extended family so that the children could not understand the conversation. This added to Jerry's fears that his mother had negative thoughts of him and kept them hidden. Susan was subjected to the same treatment, but somehow she seemed to be far less troubled by the rigidity of the household. Jerry's sister, as an adult, described their mother as warm and loving, devoted to husband and children, and as having a wide circle of friends and activities. It was Jerry's own opinion, substantiated somewhat by others outside the family, that his sister used a great deal of denial about the traumas of their childhood.

Jerry's father was rarely involved with his children, never attended a school function for them, and viewed an "A" in schoolwork as standard, without praise, while even a "B+" elicited inquiry as if it were a lamentable failure. Jerry's father had grown up in an immigrant German family of six children. He worked as a high city official in the small town where the family lived. It seemed to Jerry that his father was accustomed to being obeyed without question.

SESSIONS AND COURSE OF TREATMENT

Jerry presented himself in his sessions as a thoughtful and caring person, invariably asking about the well-being of his therapist as the first transaction of each session. These inquiries seemed genuine and caring, although they sometimes covered angry feelings that might burst forth. As mentioned earlier, aggressive statements were sometimes directly expressed to the analyst, in conjunction with proclamations that Jerry wanted to be "totally honest." Expressions of "I want to hit/kick/get you!" were more the norm, but sometimes "I want to fuck you!" would replace these others. The analyst did not experience these expressions as frightening or threatening, perhaps because they were contextualized in Jerry's apparent concern to reveal himself. Moreover, they seemed to be triggered by some thought of his (Jerry's) own inadequacy, which would then quickly produce a sense of envy of the analyst's presumed superiority. This anger manifested itself later in therapy as complaints about the analyst not "doing enough for" Jerry.

An early and significant interaction in group psychotherapy reflected the same aggressive and sexual theme. An older and more financially successful man in the group made friendly and supportive remarks to Jerry in an early session. Other group members seemed to validate the genuine quality of the older man's empathic response to Jerry. Jerry abruptly broke the feeling of empathy with the assertion, "I want to put my penis in you!" The older man recoiled; and for the remaining few months that he was in the group, he made no further approach to Jerry, although he was never overtly critical of Jerry.

Soon after entering group therapy, Jerry became the "junior therapist." He consistently asked people for their emotional responses and pushed them to be self-revealing and to "play by the rules" of group interaction. Another male member of the group, a man with many hysterical features, frequently attacked Jerry for "trying to control the group," once even challenging him to step out to the parking lot and settle their differences with a fist fight. Although nothing came of the challenge, Jerry was clearly frightened. Jerry also had some openly aggressive interchanges with women, but nothing that was disruptive.

After Jerry had been in the group more than a year, a new woman entered who, unknown to the therapist, had had a brief sexual relationship with Jerry several years before. She had subsequently married. They both revealed this history to the group in her initial session and felt that it was no barrier to their being honest in their interactions as fellow group members. She expressed pleasant memories of their dating and stated that both then and now she experienced Jerry as a warm and caring person. Jerry had felt the same way about her.

Jerry's major way of relating to the group was "right" in the letter but not the spirit of the law. His frequent criticisms of others' lack of self-disclosure were gradually perceived as judgmental. Other members frequently observed that Jerry was trying to be the therapist. Dr. Hall neither intervened nor interpreted these interactions, largely restricting himself to facilitating group process and reflection. Gradually the group's perception of Jerry shifted. He made no further hostile or sexual remarks to men in the group. The unacknowledged rivalry with the man who had challenged him to fight transformed into a (mostly) mutually respectful relationship. With increasing self-reflection, it seemed as if Jerry's initial identity as "unacknowledged therapist," mixed with over-solicitousness and hyperresponsibility for others, shifted to an identity of a regular group member able to "stand up for himself" without threats of physical aggression or psychological attacks on others.

In his individual sessions, therapeutic work centered on understanding interpersonal relations and the integration of dream interpretation. Jerry's dreams usually contained images of people he knew or persons who resembled those of daily life. Only rarely were his dreams strange, unfamiliar, mythological, or bizarre. In one, Jerry was plotting with other male students to murder his shop teacher, perhaps for money. At the last minute, just before a classmate was to shoot the teacher in the head with a homemade gun, Jerry decided to tell the teacher of the plot, but he was very frightened and woke up with anxiety. Jerry associated the dream to his father spending time in his woodworking shop rather than with Jerry and his sister and to his own anger about this. He spoke of a workbench his father had built for him, a bench appraised at more than a thousand dollars. But he dismissed his father's gift by saying "He only built it for me because he liked to build things like that—and he built a better one for himself." This workbench, which was still in the home of Jerry's mother, was eventually used in the therapy as an interpretative symbol of his father attempting to relate to Jerry, to give him something valuable, rejected by Jerry with rationalizations that destroyed the meaning of the gift.

Near the same time, Jerry dreamed that he was thinking about fly-fishing again (something his father had taught him to do). Then he was fishing on a river and caught a small fish, but then on the next try, he caught a large fish of 60 to 100 pounds. He landed the fish and was looking for something to kill it with but didn't have the correct tools. Since he did not want the fish to suffocate in the air and die painfully, he put its head in shallow water. He could see the gills work. He was afraid he would become attached to the fish and that it would then be difficult to kill it. The scene changed, and he and the fish were lying by a campfire talking. He felt warmth and affection for the fish.

In a dream occurring about 2 years after beginning analysis, Jerry was in a public restroom when he noticed a man who reminded him very much of his father. He approached the man and asked to be hugged, saying that it was something his father had never done. The man politely and kindly refused Jerry's request. Jerry found in the dream a message that his desires for affection from a substitute father were inappropriate and intrusive, but not bad. His homosexual fears seemed to diminish following this dream and its working through in treatment.

In a later dream, the image of Jerry's actual father appeared. In this dream, Jerry was in his mother's house, sleeping in his sister's bed (where he now slept when visiting his mother, since his own former room had been converted into an office). His father, whom he knew to be dead, entered the room. He noticed that the left lens of his father's glasses was darkened, while the right lens was normal and clear. He rose and embraced his father, but as he did so, he began to feel himself floating upward into the air. Afraid that he, too, was dying, Jerry experienced anxiety, and the dream ended. He took the dream to mean that if he clung too closely to anger or desire for his deceased father (or to wishes for love he had not received), he might "die"—that is, might miss living his own life because of yearning for a different type of fathering experience than he had had as a child.

As a result of this dream, Jerry contacted a former member of his psychotherapy group, a priest, and participated with the priest in a mass for his father. The objective was to facilitate the process of "letting go" of his father. Jerry was not Catholic, but the ritual had a profound calming effect on him. He later dreamed that he was with the priest (John), who had helped to construct a tall structure, perhaps with the help of Jerry. There were two parallel circular rings of boards set some distance apart on a central, circular core. Because the upper boards were laid at right angles to the lower ones, when looked at from the upper circle, where John and Jerry were lying, they made a pattern of crosses. John contacted Jesus. Jesus had been sleeping, but told the priest that he, John, had now become "his own symbol," which suggested to Jerry that Father John was now "his own man," not simply a man in the generic role of priest.

A dream late in therapy showed Jerry as a Wild-West-type Indian pursued by cowboys. The scene changed and Jerry was to be executed, with two women at hand to assist. They neither approved nor disapproved of his execution, but they wanted to help him do it in a painless manner. He was frightened, but somehow the execution seemed the result of "due process." It was ordered by a "higher court" or some other authority.

During the course of his analysis, Jerry was involved in a number of relationships with women, none of them eventuating in long-term bonding. In one of these he dealt responsibly with a triangular situation. In another, he acted with poorer judgment. He established a sexual relationship with a woman whom he liked, but whom he knew he would

not marry. The woman probably wanted greater commitment. She tended
Jerry initially by cooking very elaborate meals for him, but when her life
became more complicated she simplified the meals—something Jerry
took as a sign that he was less important to her. He finally spoke with her
about this in a way that lacked concern for her feelings, and subsequently, she began to avoid contact with him. She soon ended the
relationship over the telephone, hanging up on him as soon as she had
said it was over. Jerry had limited empathy for her, experiencing only his
own feelings of disappointment and humiliation.

His relationship with his former wife remained cordial, although
they interacted primarily through their children. Jerry recognized a
similarity in his responses to the daughter (who seemed not to appreciate
his financial support) and his lack of understanding for his girlfriend
(who stopped cooking elaborate meals).

Three years into his treatment, Jerry planned a camping and
mountain-climbing trip with a male cousin who he knew was homosexual. He had some anxiety that they were to sleep in the same tent. He
and his cousin talked about sexual matters frankly, and Jerry was
relieved that he found no sexual impulse toward the cousin. Their joint
adventure in climbing a rather impressive peak in Colorado became a
symbol for Jerry of his being able to achieve masculine goals, free of his
concern about homosexual feelings. The homosexual fantasies by now
seemed clearly linked in his mind with some unconscious attempt at
repair and restitution of the image of his father.

An elderly neighbor woman died soon after this camping trip.
During the last weeks of her life, Jerry was one of the few persons to
continue to visit her. In fact, he had a supportive visit with her the day
before her death, later telling his therapist "I hope I don't die alone like
that, and I hope you don't either." This remark seemed to reveal a more
stable and sympathetic attitude toward the therapist as a person rather
than a transferential "object."

The most important contact in the neighborhood, however, was
"Mr. F." During Jerry's daily jogging, he often saw Mr. F. tending his
garden. At times Mr. F. asked Jerry in for coffee, which he served in old
cracked cups. In most respects, Mr. F. was a socially unpleasant
person, wearing soiled and smelly clothing, his shirt sometimes stained
with tobacco juice. Most people in the neighborhood shunned Mr. F.,
but Jerry developed a friendship with him. What most impressed Jerry
was the manner in which Mr. F. loved his wife, who was confined to a
nursing home. Each day Mr. F. would visit his wife, often fixing her food
from home. When his wife died, Mr. F. shared his grief with Jerry, and
perhaps with no one else. Jerry admired the depth of relationship Mr. F.
felt for his invalid wife. When Mr. F. himself died some months later,

Jerry was one of the mourners. In his unlikely friendship with Mr. F., Jerry seemed to experience a way of relating to unacceptable parts of himself and of responding to human problems more maturely.

When Jerry spoke of the past it was most often about his father who, he felt, had not sufficiently cared for him. With time he began to attribute his present lack of a stable sense of masculinity to his father's distance, linking both his homosexual thoughts and his ambivalent kiss/kick attitude toward his therapist to paternal emotional deprivation. About 4 years into treatment, a long dream ended with Jerry using an ax to trim a log into an hexagonal shape. Dr. O. (a retired theology professor whom he greatly admired) was there and said "To have grace, you need to kill the father." This startling comment seemed to cut through the constant ambivalence about the father, projected onto the analyst as well as members of the group. Jerry contacted Dr. O. and arranged a visit with him. The content of the interview was straightforward and insightful. Jerry appreciated the sense of making personal contact with this man whom he had admired.

An example of a dream image especially important to Jerry was a dog figure that had spikes sticking out from its body, somewhat like thick spines. In the dream the dog image belonged to a woman who was described as "the Devil's daughter," although she was casting a spell to protect Jerry from the "real" Devil. Jerry did a great deal of work on the image of this dog, sketching it and reading about the symbolic meaning of dogs. The dream in which the dog figure appeared was long and complex, as were most of Jerry's dreams. At the beginning of the dream, Jerry is talking to the owner of a theater about doing some writing. Jerry is told to meet the owner inside, taking an elevator to reach the theater. There are other people in the elevator, and it moves in an odd manner— first up, then to the side, then further up—opening onto a "private" part of the theater, which resembles a very "ritzy" apartment. This private part of the theatre has a sinister feeling about it. The main room is a large bedroom 20 feet square with a large bed on an elevated platform. The elevator operator (who is male) begins transforming pillows on the bed through manipulating controls; the pillows become boxes of different sizes. It is like a performance and Jerry applauds. Then two men are having breakfast. They look like mobsters. Outside there is a man who needs help with luggage or strange shapes. Jerry and a woman offer to help with the luggage. At this point, one of the two breakfasting men comes near, quietly concealing a hand gun. The dream then transforms into a pursuit, with Jerry running through something like train station passageways in New York. Someone is right behind him. He gets back inside, hides in a closet near the doorway, and the pursuing man begins looking for him. Jerry makes pretend noises of a gun and the man begins writhing as if actually hit by a bullet. Jerry's aggression becomes stronger, and he hits the man on the head; however as Jerry becomes more aggressive so does his male opponent. Jerry's defense is clearly best with the "pretend" gun.

At this point there is a girl, about 20, in a bathroom nearby. She takes things from a cabinet. One is a statue of an animal like a dog used in religious ceremonies. It appears to be African in style. The girl says that her father is the Devil and she is looking for ways to defeat him. She places the figure of the dog to face the direction Jerry believes her father to be located. Jerry becomes terrified and makes a cross with his arms as a protective gesture. The figure of the dog is 18 inches tall, carved of wood with some 15 or so spikes, each 5 inches long, coming from its body. The body itself is white, but there are traces of red on the tips of the spikes. It is male and fierce.

This was an important dream for Jerry. It embodied in symbolic form many of his fears about male aggressiveness, which he felt he could counter in fantasy but only with difficulty in reality, as with the man in the group who "jokingly" asked him to fight. The final source of difficulty, the "Devil himself," is opposed not by Jerry, who is terrified, but by the "Devil's daughter," who knows how to use the aggressive dog image to undo her father.

At the time of this writing, Jerry is still in individual and group analysis. Although no longer distressed by acutely ambivalent feelings about men, Dr. Hall, members of his psychotherapy group, or others in his life, he does not yet feel entirely ready to end the psychotherapy contact. He has greatly improved self-esteem, has clearly demonstrated his ability to support himself in his consulting business, and has lost much of his preoccupation with homosexual fantasies. He is dating a woman whom he is thinking of marrying. With great trepidation, he told his mother that he was living with this woman. Although his mother disapproved of his living with a woman before marrying, she affirmed her love for him. Encouraged by her acceptance, he also told her how much he had disliked the enemas she had given him when he was a child. His mother explained that enemas were what she had thought were necessary to maintain his health. She was sorry if that had hurt him. Perhaps she had been wrong.

Jerry has come to a greater acceptance and understanding of himself and exhibits a greater tolerance for his own problems. There is much less aggression and yearning toward the past and his parents. Simultaneously he appears to be much closer to sustaining intimacy with a woman and making a successful remarriage.

☆7☆

Twelve Lenses
of Subjectivity:
Interpretations of Jerry

As is typical of most cases of psychotherapy, this one has many portals of entry. Because our subject is subjectivity, we organize our interpretations by the invariants of agency, coherence, continuity, and emotional arousal as these can be understood through different theoretical and clinical lenses. What we intend with this chapter is to show how the issue of subjectivity, and its attendant topics, illuminates clinical work. Moreover, we hope that our constructivist orientation will encourage us and our readers to move away from the metaphor of self as a place or a location and toward experiencing it as a strategy or a way a person goes on being a self-recognized unity.

Our purpose here is to illustrate the usefulness of the lens of self psychology in understanding the underlying meaning and/or psychopathology in the case presented. We do not intend to review any treatment strategies or decisions. We would not pretend to know how other therapists, trained in the different models that follow, would actually work with Jerry. Some of the theoretical lenses (e.g., object relations and Freudian psychoanalysis) through which we will examine Jerry are intimately connected with treatment approaches. Obviously, we are not assuming that a clinician using such an approach would have acted to handle Jerry in the same way he was treated by Dr. Hall in Jungian analysis.

In Chapter 8 we examine aspects of the clinical material—for instance, the progress of the actual transference issues—that are excluded here because we are using the case hypothetically to apply various theories of subjectivity.

FREUD, FAIRBAIRN, AND KOHUT

Freud's contributions to the psychology of subjectivity are broadly significant for our contemporary understanding of self and yet somewhat unclear because of Freud's lack of a specific construct of self. Freud almost single-handedly opened up the questions of unconscious motivations, adaptive strategies, and narrative structures of individual history that have preoccupied depth psychologists since the beginning of this century. Although Freud modified many of his models over the course of his own intellectual development, he retained the idea of conflict as the central theme of subjectivity. Fairbairn, a Scottish psychoanalyst who was strongly influenced by Melanie Klein, also emphasized the centrality of conflict in subjective organization. Fairbairn was a prominent contributor to the "British School" of psychoanalysis, also known as the object relations school (see Greenberg & Mitchell, 1983, for a complete account). As we will see, Fairbairn's structure or model for subjective development incorporates the organization of conflicting desires as a major motive force. Kohut, a Viennese psychoanalyst who became an American psychoanalyst, founded his own psychoanalytic school, now called Self Psychology. Kohut postulated a separate line of development of the self, one that deemphasizes conflict and stresses function and structure instead. These three psychoanalytic theorists cover a range of treatment strategies and models for impingements on agency, coherence, continuity, and emotional arousal.

Looking first to Freud, we recognize the theme of opposing drives, motives, and processes in both the topographical model of conscious/ perception, preconscious, and unconscious motive forces and the structural model of ego, superego, and id sub-personalities. Similarly, the opposing drives of eros (life) and thanatos (death), of love and aggression, of ego and object cathexes are all examples of the general premise that conscious awareness is an achievement or striving to resolve and mediate conflicts. Only after the publication of *Beyond the Pleasure Principle* in 1920 did Freud turn his attention specifically to the idea of mastery of conflict as the means of ego development. Particularly within his work on the structural model (*Ego and Id*, 1923, and *Inhibitions, Symptoms and Anxiety*, 1926), Freud envisioned the ego as the active, executive function of personality—as the specifically conscious activity of personal agency with its defensive structuring. Defense mechanisms such as displacement, condensation, and repression had been a part of Freudian theory from its earliest formulation, but these had not specifically been connected with the idea of mastery.

The idea that we develop consciousness through *actively* repeating (and attempting to control) what has been *passively* endured or suffered is the key concept for the process of ego development. The fundamental formulation or psychoanalytic principle of "Where it was, I shall become" (or "Where id was, ego shall be") is an extension of this principle of mastery in the sense that a developing person comes to feel progressively more responsible for her/his life and the meanings constructed from it. Simultaneously, a person comes to recognize what the limits of personal responsibility are, both in terms of the accidents and happenings of fate and in terms of the opportunities presented by luck or privilege. The intersection of neurotic *repetition compulsion* and healthy *mastery* in the neurotic individual is the arena for psychoanalytic treatment and the process of ego development in general. Active repetition of what one has passively suffered *may* become a compulsion to act out (on others and the world) or act in (on oneself) various aspects of one's powerlessness and fears from childhood. Each such occasion of repetition compulsion also provides an opportunity for active mastery if the unconscious motives can be known, understood, and controlled.

Freud's psychosexual stages of development, published first in *Three Essays on the Theory of Sexuality* (1953a/1900) provide a developmental continuum on which the drama of mastery is enacted. The *oral* period is roughly the first year of life, when the infant experiences tension between nurturant pleasures and fearful needs or overwhelming anxieties. Basic survival needs for food and security are primary, connecting the infant to the mother and resulting in mastery of reality testing or the ability to distinguish hallucinatory fantasy (e.g., of the breast) from reality. The *anal* period is from about 2 to 3 years of age and involves conflicts between the child's desire to submit to and be protected by the parents and the parents' dominance of the child's body and movement. The child's desires (e.g., to be approved, loved, and physically active) frequently seem in opposition to the parents' desires (e.g., to restrict and discipline the child for its own protection). The healthy outcome of this period is the mastery of basic autonomy or the ability to differentiate one's own body and physical movements from the pressures of authority figures while neither wholly capitulating to nor devaluing those in authority. The *phallic or Oedipal* period occurs from about 3 to 4 or 5 years of age. This phase of development is the basis of what is known as the "conflict theory" of Freudian psychoanalysis. It focuses on the child's fantasies of romantic love with the parents and how these are threatened by the aggressions of parental discipline and power/size. The child, now loving its parents as people (rather than as part-aspects of people, such as breast or voice), wants to identify with one or both parents in order to embody the power and meaning of their authority and sexuality. This Oedipal child is also aware of basic structural body differences and knows, for example, that males have penises and females do not; that females bear babies and males do not. Aware of the greater strength and power of the parents, the child experiences a conflict in its own feelings: to possess singularly the parent of the opposite sex and to obey completely the dictates of the parental powers. A healthy outcome of this period is the mastery of this conflict through the renouncing of romantic love for the opposite-sexed parent and identifying with the strengths and values of the same-sexed parent. Resolution of the Oedipal conflict—substantially different for male and female children—is the entrance into the larger culture where one must sublimate one's sexual and aggressive impulses for the aims of education and membership in society.

Less desirable outcomes of the psychosexual stages of development result in various failures of mastery and compulsions to repeat or reenact aspects of failed development that may be psychotic, perverse, or neurotic. The ability to achieve coherence and continuity of body-being is disrupted in failures of the oral and anal phases. Gross disabilities of personal agency are a result of failure to negotiate the anal period, and unresolved inner conflicts of personal agency are a result of failure to resolve the Oedipal conflict. Emotional arousal may be disrupted at any stage of psychosexual development, but its disruption is experienced most poignantly as a failure in oral mastery (psychotic defenses against emotions). Anal defenses (such as passive aggression) or neurotic defenses (such as repression and sublimation) are examples of efforts to master emotional arousal that are connected with the other stages.

The healthy outcome of the Oedipal conflict is the internalization or assimilation of the parental authority into oneself. This means that the child can now take an "as if" position of the parents toward its own impulses, desires, and wishes. From the point of view of the "ego ideal" or "superego," the child sees its own behaviors and desires as if it were the parent. Moreover, the developing sense of the personal agency of the ego (or "I" consciousness) includes an awareness of the conflicts between the superego standards of parental authority and the sexual/ aggressive wishes, desires, and impulses that continue to be aroused by the id within (instincts and repressed memories) and reality without.

Dreams (see Freud's *The Interpretation of Dreams*, 1900/1953a) are the disguised versions of these id products that are motivated by sexual and aggressive wishes. The "dream-thoughts" or "latent" dream is an unconscious wish or impulse that is unacceptable to both the superego (or censorship of the preconscious) and the ego. The transformation or

"dream-work" of the preconscious system of mental representation results in a "manifest" dream that has been disguised through condensation, displacement, secondary revision (narrative form), and symbolization. Dreams are essentially useless to the waking ego except as psychic
by-products of instinctual release, unless a person makes a corrective
psychoanalytic interpretation. Through free association (speaking whatever comes to mind from the dream motifs), a person may learn to
explore unconscious or latent dream content in a way that clarifies the
conflicts of the psyche, conflicts that the ego attempts to master through
imposing both reality-testing and superego injunctions.

Jerry presents an "anal character structure" that is marked by
limited autonomy, disturbing ambivalence about authority figures, and
occasional oppositional behavior such as outbursts of rage. From his
personal memories, Jerry identifies especially his disgust for the enemas
his mother administered and suggests that he was traumatized by her
abusive methods of discipline, the beatings with a rubber hose. His
obsessive concern with various details (such as personal mannerisms
and politeness) serves him well when he is doing technical writing or
consulting but is less attractive when he attempts to control his fellow
group members (to keep them to the rules) or to tally up whether his
woman friend is giving him "fair returns" for his investment in her. The
aggression he expresses against his therapist—displaced from anal
fantasies of the mother's punishments—is quickly undone and rational-
ized as "truth-telling," as a way of either soothing his superego demands
on himself, or placating his more primitive fears of the retaliatory parent.
Jerry's ambivalent kick/kiss attitude is particularly manifested toward
male authority figures, raising the question as to whether aspects of his
conflicts with authority figures are more Oedipal than pre-Oedipal. This
would mean that he desires the love and attentions of a fatherly figure,
but he also feels extremely competitive and envious of the power and
sexuality of that figure.

Many of Jerry's fantasies and dreams seem to reveal a classic
Oedipus complex—the unresolved struggle to defeat the father and
possess (perhaps dominate) the mother. Jerry's perception of his father
as a person who wanted to be obeyed "without question" and his
homosexual fantasies and his sexual threats to other men (aggressive in
nature, as they are) are probably greater evidence, however, that his
primary disturbances *are* anal with some Oedipal overlay.

The dream of Jerry's execution by a "higher court" suggests the
punitive type of superego associated more with the anal than the Oedipal
stage. Jerry's constant undoing of his own aggressive moves and his fear
of entering into the larger corporation to compete for his future are
further indicators of anal struggles. Longing for fusion with the father

may be the origin of the dream wish expressed in the embrace of the dead father and his subsequent fear of dying in that embrace. The dream of planning to murder the male shop teacher is only a thinly disguised murderous impulse against the authority of Dr. Hall—who is now the teacher of the "work bench lesson" (good-enough father). Having another person point the gun, using a pretend gun in another dream, and frequently being on the "victim" side of aggressive chases are all displacements of his own aggression onto others. Additionally, these factors probably indicate Jerry's fundamental feeling of being hopelessly castrated or disempowered by the mother's destructive interventions, unprotected by any powerful father. Jerry identifies more with being a good/bad little boy—seeing the big parental figures as the Others—and less with being a contender for relationships and work in an adult male sphere.

Trauma in the anal stage of development probably interfered with a healthy sense of personal agency in young Jerry. Moreover, adapting to severe and punitive parents, Jerry learned to defend his ego through such anal defenses as passive–aggression, identification with the aggressor, acting out, and undoing. Displacement, repression, intellectualization, and sublimation are more mature defenses that Jerry has developed through a partial ability to cope with some Oedipal conflicts. His devaluation of his mother and his fears of aggressive or phallic women seem to impede the full blossoming of Oedipal struggles. In Jerry's ongoing identification with Dr. Hall as the Oedipal father, Jerry has become more and more capable of taking on Oedipal struggles such as feeling empowered to confront his mother and to identify with being a fully sexual man (with his new partner). Being able to experience Dr. Hall as both remote and loving, as both protective and challenging, Jerry can unify the experiences of being male in both "strong" and "weak" forms.

Fairbairn's particular contribution to psychoanalytic object relations theory is the assertion that libido or the thrust of psychological attention is object-seeking (i.e., relational in nature) rather than simply discharge-seeking (i.e., conditioned by pleasure). He thus focuses attention directly on the interface between interpersonal relationships and intrapsychic dynamics. His work follows especially the influence of Melanie Klein, who defined two major developmental tasks of early subjectivity: moving beyond the "paranoid–schizoid" construction of earliest psychic reality and then beyond the "depressive" construction of loss and destruction, the emotional results of one's own aggressive needs. Achievement of the depressive position permits people to experience themselves and others in stable (continuous, coherent), but ambivalent (good/bad) terms. Failure to achieve this developmental perspective results in lifelong difficulties with ambivalence and instability in intimate relationships. Failure to resolve the depressive position results in lifelong problems with feelings of guilt and desires to make reparations (for one's own aggressions) for the nature of one's own needs.

In a series of articles and books, Fairbairn (1952, 1954) gradually evolved a model of intrapsychic conflict that paralleled and extended Freud's model of ego, id, and superego, integrating Klein's understanding of the effects of paranoid–schizoid and depressive images on ego functioning. Fairbairn conceived of three states of personal agency or ego-consciousness: central, libidinal, and antilibidinal. These three functional types of subjective being were correlated with three types of intrapsychic images: ideal, exciting, and rejecting. The neutral or central desire for conflict-free subjective being was matched to an intrapsychic image of an ideal or neutral figure (object). The libidinal or aroused desire for stimulating contact was matched to an image of an exciting figure. The antilibidinal or anxious, inhibitory desire was matched to an image of a rejecting or threatening figure. These three functional states of personal being are both structures and processes of psychic experience. They result in formulated images and expectations of self and other. Defenses of each effectively split them off from the others, so that early life experiences tend to be discontinuous in these three states of subjectivity. The vicissitudes of these states correspond to both the intrapsychic nature of a particular person and the experiences of early interpersonal relationships, especially those in the earliest pre-Oedipal periods.

Jerry's recent romantic relationship is an illustration of a pre-Oedipal organization within his current experience of subjectivity, as per Fairbairn. Jerry first perceived his woman friend as an exciting object within an aroused state of libidinal desire, but when she (under her own pressures from job and educational commitments) failed to perform according to his image (she stopped cooking elaborate meals), Jerry projected into her the rejecting antilibidinal object and perceived himself to be in a state of inhibition or depletion. He was unable to do anything about this because it was "her fault," not under his control. This is evidence that Jerry has not successfully resolved the paranoid–schizoid perspective and uses psychological "splitting" as a defense against the terror of abandonment. When his friend behaves in a nongratifying way, Jerry immediately projects into her the rejecting parent, unable to integrate the good/bad aspects of the Other. Jerry broke up the relationship abruptly and then returned to a neutral, central sense of personal agency—unable to "figure out" what had happened.

In Jerry's dream of the shop teacher, we see a similar pattern of instability. Jerry (in an antilibidinal state) participates in planning the murder of the mother/father–therapist (the rejecting object). His identity shifts to the central–neutral state that opposes the friend who has the gun (who now is the rejecting Other). In waking life Jerry's states of personal subjectivity shift around within this tripartite dynamic without his recognizing the sense of conflict between them. This kind of splitting results in discontinuous and incoherent experiences of self, a state hypothesized by Fairbairn and Klein to be like infancy and early life in the paranoid–schizoid position.

Although Jerry is not functioning primarily at this early stage of development, we can see that many aspects of his relationships with women/Mother are organized by libidinal (need/arousal) and anti-libidinal (fear/inhibition) states of ego consciousness. As we said earlier, the Oedipal identification with an ambivalently loved, admirable father–therapist has seemed to provide a necessary strengthening of Jerry's central–neutral ego consciousness. Now Jerry is beginning to integrate the splits in the Mother imago (exciting/threatening) that probably interfered with his ability to move on developmentally. Evidence for this is his recent ability to sustain himself and face the potential aggression of his actual mother in confronting her about his enemas and telling her about his new live-in relationship. In understanding her responses, he seems able to have ambivalent feelings about her, rather than grossly split states of being.

Whereas Fairbairn stresses the value of ambivalence in psychological relationships, Kohut stresses the value of idealization. Kohut (1971, 1977, 1984) postulates a separate line of development of the self—much like the neutral or central ego of Fairbairn—and deemphasizes conflict. Infants go through two stages that are critical to the formation of healthy self-confidence: in the first stage there is an overwhelming need to display competences and be admired; in the second stage there is a need to sustain an idealized image of at least one parent and to experience a feeling of merger with that image. In the state of complete dependence on parents (as powerful and grand figures in the child's life), the developing person forms both a "grandiose" self (powerful and important) and an "idealized" parent (who is omniscient and omnipotent). The grandiose self is both a necessary product of identification with this powerful parental image and a sufficient basis for later development of realistic self-love.

The gradual evolution out of narcissistic preoccupations with one's own grandiosity is negotiated primarily through the empathic responses of the idealized parents. This empathic responding includes the parents' ability to love and to discipline the developing child in a just way, and to mirror that child's abilities in a useful (i.e., realistic) way. The way the child negotiates such experiences as fear of the loss of parental love depends a great deal on the parents' empathy and their abilities to mirror and to discipline adequately.

The parents function as the earliest "self-objects"—the figures who provide us with the ability to maintain self-esteem and confidence in our abilities. These figures are called self-objects because their representations include elements both of one's experiences of subjectivity (similar to Fairbairn's ego states) and one's construction of another (similar to the corresponding object-images). Self-objects are neither entirely self nor entirely other. Disturbances in early self-object relationships may create narcissistic wounds in one's ability to sustain later agency, coherence, continuity, and arousal. These wounds appear as deficits in the ability to sustain subjective being, especially self-love. What results in such a case is the experience of fragments of love (sexual fantasies) rather than whole love, or fragments of confident assertiveness (hostile fantasies) rather than self-assertion.

When the empathic relationship with the idealized parents is secure and realistic, there is initially little to distinguish the projection of idealized self-object from the actual parent. The natural inevitable small failures in parental empathy or opportunities for idealization provide the means for modulating the grandiose self and the idealized self-objects. If the relationship with the idealized parents is disturbed—by the parents' inability to be empathic in gross or subtle ways—then there is an experience of deprivation that is usually felt as a lack of a basic sense of meaning. Like an experience of "loss of soul," a major empathic failure results in a profound inability to cohere as a vital person. Deficits in the fundamental construction of self are considered by Kohut to be more central to psychopathology than the experience of subjective conflict described in Freud's model of ego, id, superego. As Kohut (1984) says,

> self psychology considers the structural and functional deficiencies of the patient's self as the primary disorder. . . . whereas traditional analysis saw the contents of conflicts as the primary disorder and focused on it. (p. 29)

The sexual and aggressive impulses that Freud characterized as products of the id or unconscious—making demands on the ego that conflict with reality and superego ideals—are for Kohut indicators of failed pre-Oedipal development. They are a function of the fragmentation of early desires to love and be competent. From Kohut's perspective, incestuous desires for sexual involvement with parents or parental figures are symptoms of pre-Oedipal disturbances in a person's ability to achieve and sustain personal agency, coherence, continuity, and emotional arousal. In the place of an experience of individual subjectivity, such a person strives to experience self through grandiose fantasies of power, suffering, fame, or achievement, or alternately desires to possess others who appear in an idealized light that promises to bestow special resources or strengths.

In the case of Jerry, we have an impression that both of his parents were overtly critical and even harsh in their perceptions of Jerry's failures. From Jerry's memories he believes that his father always failed to praise or notice his achievements; he was ruled by standards that were unrelated to the actual abilities of children. His mother intruded punitively to humiliate Jerry when she should have disciplined him. Moreover, it is apparent that Jerry has failed to idealize his parents because he cannot desist in his criticisms of them. Like many survivors of empathic failure in childhood, Jerry's self-esteem seems predicated on a negative view of the parent. Had he been able to idealize and then surrender the idealization, Jerry would be more forgiving of parental faults and others' current empathic failures.

Not only his therapist but many other male authority figures (e.g., Dr. O.) have become self-objects for Jerry. Dr. Hall is the target of Jerry's criticisms of perceived failures, especially in what Jerry sees to be Dr. Hall's inability to empathize with Jerry's torture at the hands of his father. (Jerry is resistant to accepting any positive valuation of his father, especially when Dr. Hall implies that the workbench, and other signs of affection, might be indicators that his father loved him.) On the other hand, Jerry does idealize Dr. Hall and desires a merger with him. Jerry's desire to merge with the idealized self-object is evident in his becoming the "junior therapist" in his group. This merger made him the object of his fellow members' indignation and, alas, became a display of his own dysfunction. Another event in the group provided a chance opportunity for empathic mirroring, however. The arrival of his former friend and lover, now married to another man, was a surprise to Jerry and everyone else. Jerry experienced his mature self mirrored by her positive memories and her warm reacquaintance with him, accompanied nonetheless with the realistic boundary of her marriage to someone else. Since her integration into the group, Jerry has been able to maintain his self-esteem and to stop the merger identification with an idealized version of Dr. Hall. In individual treatment, Jerry has gradually internalized a more realistic image of himself both as a confident, loving man and as an angry, and sometimes exacting, critic of others.

HARRÉ, PIAGET, AND BOWLBY

Philosopher Harré, researcher and theorist Piaget, and psychiatrist and researcher Bowlby may seem to be an unlikely trio, but they have important and somewhat overlapping contributions to make to a theory of self. Harré's account of the self as secondary to the person, Piaget's action-oriented dialectic of assimilation and accommodation, and Bowlby's theory of human instinct and what he terms "adaptive working models" have been essential backdrops to our explanations of a Jungian constructivism throughout.

Introducing Harré, we recall that he asserts that experience and beliefs about "self" are secondary to that of "person." That is, the invariants of personal being (agency, coherence, continuity, and emotional arousal) are first experienced as aspects of embodied being, as aspects of being a person. They are later organized into a theory (or coherent construction) of one's own subjectivity, a self. He says,

> Necessarily all human beings who are members of moral orders are persons, social individuals, but the degree of their psychological individuality, their personal being, I take to be contingent. (Harré, 1989, p. 388)

Psychological individuality, the experience of being an individual person, is contingent on the practices of family, group, or tribe in regard to the type and meaning of selfhood a person constructs. As Harré (1989) demonstrates, there is a wide range of types of selves, illustrated by the Copper Eskimos' "collective selves" (e.g., "When one weeps, they all weep; when one laughs, they all laugh." [p. 399]) on one end of the spectrum, and by the Maoris' strongly organized individuality that appears as substantialized power (e.g., *mana*) on the other. Harré contends that our typical Western self theory "seems to be located somewhere toward a midpoint of a spectrum of self-theories distinguished by the degree of emphasis on individual uniqueness, independence, and power" (p. 397).

Harré believes that the self becomes an organized theory by which a person lives her/his life and anticipates the lives of others. Such theorizing is the means by which human beings become psychological beings, according to Harré:

> Animate beings are fully human if they are in possession of a theory—a theory about themselves. It is a theory in terms of which a being orders, partitions, and reflects on its own experience and becomes capable of self-intervention and control. (1989, p. 404)

Acquiring this kind of theory is predicated on the previously acquired ability to organize oneself as a point of view and point of action that are continuous and familiar. Both consciousness and agency contribute to the organization of a life trajectory (continuity) that permits the ground-work for self ascriptions.

How do persons acquire such ascriptions? Through relationships, Harré believes. Such relationships (as between mother and child) pro-vide the images and ideals that foster the account of oneself as an individual, an account that encourages us to organize experiences of agency, coherence, continuity, and emotional arousal into a subjective unity. Harré calls this kind of mutual self relationship a "symbiosis" and he says,

> In psychological symbiosis mothers do not talk *about* the child's wishes and emotions: they *supply* the child's wishes, needs, in-tentions, wants, and the like and interact with the child as if it had them. Psychological symbiosis is a supplementation by one person of another person's public display in order to satisfy the criteria of personhood with respect to psychological competencies and attri-butes. . . . (italics in original, 1989, pp. 414–415)

Harré believes that symbiotic relationships are ongoing over the life-span, taking place in all kinds of arenas of everyday life. The theoretical construct of an individual self is supported both through others' attribu-tions and through experiences of agency or intentionality.

According to psychologists Lewis, Sullivan, Stanger, and Weiss (1989), Pipp, Fischer, and Jennings (1987), and others, the identifica-tion of self as one's own specific subjective unity is achieved roughly in the latter half of the second year of life. What Lewis et al. have called the "secondary emotions"—those that are self-conscious and self-evaluative (such as pride and embarrassment)—emerge and can be witnessed in a child only after a referential self has been experienced. Lewis has operationally defined self-referential behavior as the ability of the child to look at its image in a mirror and to show, by pointing and touching, that the image in the mirror is located at the child's body location (p. 20). With few exceptions, children will accomplish this self-referential action some time between 18 and 24 months and "there is only weak evidence to indicate any direct effect of early emotional life on the referential self" (Lewis et al., p. 20). Lewis et al. conclude then that "all" children (except in cases of the most traumatic arrests) develop the ability to refer to themselves as locations in a body.

How does this material apply to Jerry's case? First, we can assume that psychotherapy, both individual and group, is an occasion for psy-chological symbiosis in which "people complete inadequate social and psychological beings through public symbiotic activity, particularly in talking for each other" (Harré, 1989, p. 415). Although therapeutic discourse usually occludes "talking for" another person, it nevertheless is an effort to supplement another's personal being, often specifically in regard to the aspect of individual agency. In terms of agency or intentionality, group members and Dr. Hall function to show Jerry (Dr. Hall shows him by not reacting, and group members by reacting) that *he is responsible* for his moods and fantasies, his wishes and fears. When Dr. Hall does not react to the verbalized threats to hit or kick, Jerry has an opportunity to review or reflect on his behavior, to perhaps *deduce* that Dr. Hall is not afraid of the threat, and hence is taking the spoken threat *to be a fantasy*. By contrast, peers (such as the members of the therapy group) will hold him accountable for his verbalizations. Through these contrasting experiences, Jerry is able to supplement his theory of personal agency and to include the idea that he is responsible and accountable for his moods and wishes when he *expresses* these in the presence of other people.

Diagnostically, Harré's theory provides the opportunity to review whether an individual experiences difficulties in aspects of personal being, in self-construction and maintenance, and/or in reflecting on the self (i.e., the "backward glance"). In the case of Jerry, we can easily see that Jerry is capable of sustaining an ordinary sense of agency, coherence, continuity, and emotional arousal under most conditions and relationships of daily life (i.e., in nosological terms, he is not psychotic).

In specific conditions of relating to authoritative men and women, however, Jerry appears to have difficulty in maintaining a viable sense of himself as an agent. Under certain conditions, he appears to recreate the symbiosis of the parental relationship with both parents, who apparently considered it their firm responsibility to maintain order and discipline. Their symbiosis with Jerry was not one in which Jerry was encouraged to be a fully agentic person. When Jerry worries about his ability to control his impulses, to meet the objectives of a task he already knows he can perform, and/or to trust the helpfulness of concerned others, his self theory is expressed in childish terms with exaggerated wishes and fears being taken literally.

Dr. Hall's assessment of "chronic low-grade . . . depression" would fit the notion that Jerry considers himself to be helpless (i.e., not an agent) in regard to certain adult relationships and activities. Similarly the image or impression of casual youthfulness could be understood to connect with a youth or boy who is not yet fully prepared to enact his adult agency.

The *contrast* between the neutrality of an authority figure (Dr. Hall) in individual psychotherapy and the committed involvement of his peers in group psychotherapy appears to be a powerful therapeutic intervention from the point of view of Jerry's self theory. Jerry finds himself in two symbiotic situations (individual and group therapy) in which certain differences become apparent. He has to figure out why and how they are different. Why did group members react with frustration and even irritation to Jerry's "helpfulness," whereas Dr. Hall showed no apparent reaction? The evolution of Jerry's self theory is apparent in group therapy and his dreams, as the images shift and the implied meaning of his experience of himself includes more range and interest.

The psychological theory of Piaget (1926, 1932, 1936) provides another angle from which to consider Harré's notion of the secondary character of the self. Assimilation and accommodation are the dialectic components of thoughtful action in Piaget's concept of development in human life. Assimilation and accommodation are both aspects of adaptation; adaptation means roughly the ability to sustain a self-recognized unity as a person-among-persons, as a person-among-animals, and as a person-among-things. Assimilation is the more conservative side of the dialectical process; it is the activity of integrating new experiences or stimuli or data into *already existing* organizations or representations. Assimilation transforms anything *new* into something that is already familiar. Accommodation is the progressive or developmental side of adaptation; it is the activity of developing new organizations or representations when the existing ones can no longer integrate new experience.

All people come into being through biological organization or embodiment. Although organized biology is present in the human being from the start, the psychological process of development depends on the interaction of the human infant with the environment, both personal and nonpersonal. When an infant meets a "resistance" or barrier to further action (as, for example, when its sucking produces no milk), the infant attempts to assimilate or use already existing schemes of action (for example, rooting around again for the nipple, grasping with the hand, etc., depending on the age of the infant). As Overton (1990) points out, this kind of assimilation is the first confrontation with "necessity" or "reality." He says, "Necessity is the expression of integrations realized through the activity of assimilation. Possibility is the expression of differentiations realized through the activity of accommodation" (p. 19). The new possibility in the case of sucking might be to add a "complaint" or a cry to the sucking activity, communicating the distress.

Piaget (1936) develops more fully the sensorimotor origin of necessity and possibility to show how the basic action schemes of assimilation and accommodation become self-regulating systems that lead to progressively higher levels of propositional and conceptual reasoning. Just as Harré argues that the "transcendental unity" of the self is not given as a category of the human mind, Piaget argues that our understanding of logical necessity is neither a "hard-wired" product of the cerebral cortex nor a product of inductive generalizations from direct observations of "the world" (both realist arguments). Logical necessity develops rather from the patterned interactions of a person with the environment in formulating the characteristics of agency, coherence, continuity, and emotional arousal. A logical *implication* (a relation that holds between premises and conclusions: "If *p*, then *q*") develops from the necessary relationship between one situation and another. Sensorimotor action patterns (0–3 years) lead to preoperational thought forms (3–7 years), representations of self and world that are idiosyncratic and "dream-like" from an adult viewpoint. These representational forms are further organized through language and action to establish basic categories for representing time, space, causality, and the fundamentals of logic such as "and," "or," and "not"—what Piaget terms "concrete operational thought."

The full range of deductive and inductive reasoning is not present, however, until adolescence, the period when "formal thought" (11–18 years) develops. Formal thought is characterized by the ability to operate on thought structures, to reason both deductively and inductively, and to understand the antecedents and consequences of thoughts and actions. The psychological experience of "self-awareness"—in terms of the ability to understand one's motivations and to acknowledge one's responsibility—is not fully possible until one has achieved formal thought.

As we discussed earlier, Piaget has not formulated a psychological theory of the individual subject. Rather, he has revealed the structure of knowledge (representation) and perception as indications of a universal epistemic subject, the tendency to experience a self as the center of activity. Similarly, Harré (1989) wants to investigate the typical narrative uses of "I" because he assumes that such an investigation will reveal the process by which persons acquire selves. He says

> The referential aspects of the use of *I* as a theoretical term must be examined as seriously as one would the putative claim to denote something of important concepts in physics or chemistry. There are three obvious possibilities: the *self* which has no referent; its referent is the same as that of the public–collective concept *person;* or it refers to structural and dynamic features of organization of experience. (p. 410)

Naturally both Harré and Piaget have tended to endorse the last choice.

Back to Jerry, what can we see now from a Piagetian perspective? To some extent Jerry seems to confuse preoperational and operational thought. That is, Jerry responds to certain kinds of psychological "rules" (e.g., to be honest in therapy) as though they transcended time and space and the moral order of the moment. Rather than being able to experience an "as if" quality in his images of Dr. Hall as rule-giver or disciplinarian, Jerry experiences these images "thus so," as momentary intrusions that demand reprisal. If Jerry were fully capable of understanding the difference between the "letter" and the "spirit" of the law, he could capture in his own actions the distinction between being a participant in the group (i.e., responsible for his own behavior in terms of talking about *his* feelings and thoughts) and being a leader of the group (i.e., responsible for directing others to talk about their feelings). The ability to discriminate preoperational and concrete thought leads to a free use of metaphor in the later formal operational period.

At the beginning of treatment, Jerry seemed unable to think metaphorically. He would blurt out an aggressive impulse, but not really see it "as if." In the dream about John and Jesus, we can see his difficulty in discriminating between role (a sort of metaphor) and person. It seems as though Jerry had confused the role of priest with the *man* John. Jerry had not been able to see clearly the difference between a particular functional capacity—a *persona*—of a person, (e.g., as a priest or a therapist) that *stands for* the person in some settings and the fundamental being of that person. It is also possible that Jerry believed that his threats to Dr. Hall were "pretended" and that they could not hurt Dr. Hall because Dr. Hall was "a therapist." Because Dr. Hall experienced no direct hostility in the remarks (i.e., he *could* tell that Jerry's confusion was between preoperational and operational thought rather than between sensorimotor and operational thought, in which case Jerry might have actually hit Dr. Hall), he remained neutral. Other members of the group did not make the distinction Dr. Hall did. Similarly, when Jerry's woman friend cooked less elegant meals for him, Jerry seemed to "translate" this gesture into a concrete rejection of himself. By the time that the dream figure of Dr. O. told him "To have grace, you need to kill the father," Jerry seemed able to experience this as a metaphor, as a symbolic representation of a feeling state.

The ability to discriminate "fantasy" and "reality" is the ability to conserve the meanings of pre-operational or metaphorical thought, while reasoning logically about how and why it arose. Logical thinking, especially deductive reasoning, apparently becomes available to everyone by late adolescence under normal circumstances (according to Overton and his colleagues, 1987, who have been using a well-standardized test to measure it). Hence, the competence or capacity to use deductive and inductive reasoning is *available* ordinarily to all adults, but it is *applied* only sporadically, according to Overton et al. (1987). Depending on how an individual constructs the meaning of a particular situation, and depending on the rules of the moral order or social group, a person may or may not use formal reasoning to understand what is taking place.

We could speculate that Jerry's difficulty in reasoning about his women friends and authoritative males has to do both with the symbiotic relationships of childhood (and their influence on the development of various forms of knowledge in relation to the self) and with the losses at the present time. Jerry has sustained major losses of (1) his marriage and daughters (although not complete isolation from his daughters) and (2) his recent 2-year intimate relationship. From Bowlby's (1969) point of view, these losses could influence Jerry's ability both to concentrate on his own welfare and to form another relationship with a partner. Loss of bonded others in adulthood, whether through death or divorce, may produce an acute affective response in terms of what Bowlby calls "separation anxiety." The stages of normal separation anxiety are protest, despair, and apathy/restoration. In grief over extensive loss, people frequently remain in the stages of despair and apathy for long periods of time. Jerry's difficulties with motivation may be connected with separation anxiety, and certainly his fears about being rejected could also.

Looked at from another angle, Jerry's difficulties in relating (especially in trusting that others do not intend hostility or reprisal) can be understood as part and parcel of his "working model" in terms of Bowlby's (1986) newer conceptualization of how patterns of early bonding affect later personality development. In describing his newer propositions concerning the development of the self (as individual subjectivity) he says

> (a) that emotionally significant bonds between individuals have basic survival functions and therefore a primary status; (b) that they can be understood by postulating cybernetic systems situated within . . . each partner which have the effect of maintaining proximity or ready accessibility of each partner to the other; (c) that in order for the systems to operate efficiently each partner builds in his mind working models of self and of other, and of the patterns of interaction that developed between them. . . . (1986, p. 8)

Bowlby and his associates have identified three such working models of self and other. The first is called the pattern of *secure attachment* and is characterized by confidence, responsiveness, and helpfulness on the part of early caregivers. The self is organized as bold, comfortable, and responsive to receiving protection or assistance. The second pattern is *anxious resistant attachment* in which the caregiver may or may not be helpful when called on. Because of the uncertainty about caregiver response, the person is prone to separation anxiety and tends to be clinging and somewhat fearful or hesitant. This pattern is promoted by a parent being available and helpful on some occasions and not on others and by separations or threats of abandonment used as a means of control. The third pattern is that of *anxious avoidant attachment* in which the person has no confidence that care will be provided when needed or that she/he will be responded to helpfully. The person expects rebuff and attempts to become entirely self-reliant, living life without the support of others. This pattern results from parents constantly rebuffing the child's approaches. Extreme cases are results of repeated rejection and ill treatment and/or prolonged institutional care.

It appears that Jerry's working model is of an anxious resistant attachment. Both Jerry's mother and his father are described as parents who could be counted on "sometimes" but who demanded certain kinds of performance in order to provide care. Jerry's fearfulness about the potential for aggressive attack from others actually predisposes him to be aggressive. The "protest" or rage aspect of separation anxiety is frequently and easily triggered in people who have been punished by separation threats (e.g., "If you don't straighten out, we'll send you to the children's home"). Jerry's threats to others have the style of being "tests" or trials of others' good faith or ability to be trusted.

SULLIVAN, STERN, AND WINNICOTT

H. S. Sullivan, an interpersonal psychiatrist and theorist, is perhaps best known for his rendering of different realities or modes of adaptation—prototaxic, parataxic, and syntaxic. His theory of a "self-system" of defensive structure ("security operations") and his theory of anxiety as disintegration have been helpful in adapting Jungian psychology to a more interpersonal approach (see Young-Eisendrath, 1984, for an account of this).

Stern is a psychoanalytic psychiatrist whose major interest has been developmental psychopathology, especially the tracing of early development of the self as it may manifest in later behavior or in symptoms. Stern's theory provides a model of emergent, core, subjective, and verbal selves. Significantly, Stern's (1985) major work is related closely to Jungian analyst Fordham's (1969, 1985) theory of "de-integration" of the archetypal self. Both assert, from clinical work and infant observation, that the individuality of the self is already strongly organized at birth.

Winnicott, a British psychoanalyst and psychiatrist, was first a pediatrician and later a child analyst. He is a major contributor to the

British School of Psychoanalysis in object relations theory. Winnicott differs from Stern and Fordham by assuming a natural unity or symbiosis of infant and mother in the earliest stages of development. Winnicott is perhaps best known for his ideas of "holding environment" and "good-enough mothering" as the essential ingredients for the development of self. The good-enough mother would be optimally available and attuned to the infant's needs; she is the initial "facilitating environment" for early development. Even the most effective facilitating environment eventually fails to meet the infant's needs perfectly, and it is within this failure that personality forms. From Winnicott's perspective, the ability to play or to inhabit a "potential space" between self and other is the ability that contributes most to the development of self, as we shall see.

Let us look first at Sullivan's (1953, 1956) theory of a "self-system" that is comprised of "security operations" or defenses against anxiety. From Sullivan's viewpoint, the self-system is a defensive structure built from experience to cope with anxiety. Anxiety is a fundamentally disintegrating tension; it contrasts with the tension of needs (such as hunger, sleep, sex) that is fundamentally integrating. Anxiety does not lead to any particular action, any particular goal. Needs, on the other hand, always lead to a particular goal (to be fed, to be held, etc.), thus promoting learning. Learning is the increasing discrimination of opposites or contrasts that eventually results in "foresight," becoming the basis of consciousness. Foresight is the ability to know about the potential outcome of an action prior to taking that action; foresight provides a sense of freedom in human life.

Anxiety interferes with foresight and generally disorganizes perception and observation. Sullivan avers that anxiety—different from the tension of needs, which is inherent—is learned. Anxiety is learned interpersonally, is imitated, and is activated by the anxiety of people in the infant's life. Mothering ones, as Sullivan called the caregivers of early life, communicate anxiety through voice, gesture, and handling of the infant. Furthermore, anxiety is learned through contact with the anxious breast. When the mother is anxious, the breast, though full, will not let down milk. The infant perceives the breast to be full and assumes that it will produce, that it is to be the "good breast." When the anxious breast instead is empty or dry, the infant is confused and frustrated. What appeared to be so is not so. This is a metaphor for many later psychological difficulties.

Security operations are protective habits that develop to deal with anxiety in the interpersonal environment. An important security operation is "selective inattention," the ability to screen out certain data of experience that generally arouse anxiety when they are noticed. For example, if a mother's (frequent or angry) tears arouse anxiety in the child, later in life the witnessing of a woman crying may seem devoid of meaning or communication.

The self-system is organized into "good-me," "bad-me," and "not-me" in its earliest form. Good-me experiences are associated with the satisfaction of needs and the perception of a good-mothering one. Bad-me is associated with nonsatisfaction (frustration) and anxiety and with the perception of a bad-mothering one, a rejecting or overwhelming negative parent. Not-me experiences are completely outside of conscious awareness; they are not coherently organized; they are rooted in experiences of severe anxiety (such as when a child is shouted out, humiliated, brutalized, or abused). Severe anxiety is like a "blow to the head" and does not *mean* anything at all. It is merely disruptive to meaning and continuity. If the self-system has excessive not-me experiences, dropped out of awareness, then there is the potential of malignant psychopathology such as the psychoses and personality disorders.

The initial self-system of infancy (good-me, bad-me, and not-me) is reorganized in the childhood period (about 24–48 months in Sullivan's model). The self-system initially is *prototaxic* in infancy, based on prototypic discriminations of body states of hunger/satiation, affects of various sorts, distress/comfort, etc. In childhood, then, the self-system is re-organized as a self–other dynamism of *parataxic* meaning. Parataxic meanings arise directly from the association of experiences in emotionally charged moments. Aspects of subjective experience are associated to *each other* rather than to another meaning system. The self-system is formulated in childhood around the sense of "my body" (as myself) and all that my body does (eat, yawn, defecate, urinate, etc.). The use of language also begins in the childhood period. When language becomes fairly well organized, it provides the basis for *syntaxic* meaning or the association of one's experiences with the "objectivity" of others' experiences. The method of "consensual validation"—validation of meaning through consensus of another with oneself—is the basis of sanity in Sullivan's model and depends on language for its completion. The body-self of childhood is later replaced (in the juvenile period or school years) with an identity or sense of "myself." Chumship or friendship with same-sexed peers is the central pathway for developing the self-system in the juvenile period.

The self-system continues to be reorganized over time, until finally it includes a capacity for love and loneliness in early adulthood. Love is the ability to regard another as important as oneself (not more or less). Loneliness is the capacity to miss this other when the other is absent. Love and lust must blend in order for a person to have a truly intimate relationship with the opposite sex, the overall goal of human development (from a Sullivanian point of view). The fully human repertoire includes love, intimacy, and security with a person of the opposite sex.

> When I speak of one's finally being free to devote one's abilities to . . . whatever . . . you wish to quote as durable justification for life . . . that comes only when one has established a relationship of love in both the biologically and culturally ordained . . . sense. (Sullivan, quoted in Perry, 1981)

Because the self-system is a defense against anxiety, it is always at odds with intimacy. Especially if a "malevolent transformation" (the general communication from the elders that outsiders are not to be trusted and intend harm towards the family or self) has taken place, a child may come to be suspicious of anyone outside the family.

When a self-system is strongly organized, full of selective inattention, and especially vigilant about the trustworthiness of others, then a person is at risk for being unable to relate intimately and unable to experience what Sullivan assumed was the basis of all morality: reciprocity based on trust.

Jerry entered therapy because of persistent fears of inadequacy, fears that prevented him from returning to work in a large corporation because of vulnerability to "sudden dismissal." He was troubled by homosexual fantasies and found it difficult to maintain an intimate relationship with a woman, although he had been married. According to Sullivan (1953), anxiety in adolescence and adulthood is a direct response to lowered self-esteem. When self-esteem is threatened by real or imagined stimuli that are reminiscent of childhood (parataxic) patterns, then a person experiences anxiety and becomes more defensely organized. Anxious mothering in early life and childhood is often the origin of parataxic meanings that later threaten self-esteem. Jerry's accounts of severe beatings and enemas would likely mean that Jerry's self-system is organized with prominent bad-me and not-me dynamisms regarding his sexuality and his achievements.

Jerry's thinking and actions sometimes exhibit parataxic features when he blurts out threats or challenges that seem to be otherwise out of context. Furthermore, Jerry seems to want good-mother communications—communications of support, sustenance, praise, etc. His "invariably asking about the well-being of his therapist" is a security operation of the self in a Sullivanian context. His self-system is organized to avoid the aggressions of others, but he is the first to be aggressive in some situations (apparently when a strong authority figure appears to be powerful). From the accounts of Jerry's relationships with

women, it appears that his aggressive tendencies emerge after he becomes friendly or intimate with a woman. We can imagine that this
intimacy reactivates aspects of the early bad-mother, anxious-mother
parataxic systems. Jerry responds then by becoming defensively critical
or by distancing himself emotionally.

Sullivan observed in his clinical work that further development of
the self-system always depends on new interpersonal opportunities. He
considered personality to be the relatively enduring interpersonal relationships that characterize a human life. For Sullivan, the self develops
only through relationships, never in isolation or withdrawal. Jerry developed an increasing sense of trust through his contacts with other
group members and his neighbors and cousin. When members of the
group did not fit his parataxic distortions—such as his fear of aggressive
retaliation—then Jerry was able to reformulate aspects of the self-system
to fit new interpersonal data. On the other hand, when he perceived his
female companions as "validating" his suspicions about their dominating
or denying characteristics, Jerry continued to use parataxic distortions
and imagined them to be frightening and aggressive. Obviously the
special distinction of a therapeutic relationship is that it works to contain
and understand the aggressions of clients, whereas other interpersonal
relationships (family and friends) often cannot tolerate destructive
reenactments of parataxic distortions.

Jerry's mountain-climbing trip with his cousin proved to be an
exception. He was able to sleep next to his homosexual cousin despite
his anxieties. He and the cousin were able to communicate on a syntaxic
level of new meanings and possibilities. Jerry no longer feared that he
was homosexual because of his longing for closeness with older males.
After the trip, Jerry was able to perceive and integrate positive aspects of
other relationships in a new way.

In the dream of the Devil's dog, we see imagistic evidence of the
transformation of Jerry's self-system in regard to male aggression. In the
dream, Jerry first assumes that the male elevator operator is a magician,
that he has magic powers (perhaps this is an image of Dr. Hall). When
Jerry agrees to help the "mobster" characters who seem to be images of
"bad-me," he is attacked (one of the men has a gun) and then pursued.
When he opposes the mobster character (hits the man on the head), he
then encounters a female protagonist with a powerful dog statue. This
female figure is able to cope with the Devil father. What seems to be
expressed is a transformation of the bad-me (not male) into a good-me
(capable of initiative), who is assisted by a powerful female partner.
Jerry's bad-me self-system was frequently activated in the presence of
aggressive feelings about male authority figures; when he cooperated
with it (such as making threats to other males), he frequently got into

trouble. When he did not cooperate with it (but opposed it on the basis of his understanding), he could identify with being a powerful male himself, partnered by a powerful female.

One aspect of Stern's (1985) theory, in particular, gives us entry into why Jerry may have such difficulty trusting intimate relations with men and committing himself anew to a woman. This aspect is what Stern calls "representations of interactions that have been generalized" or RIGs (pp. 97–99 and 114–119). RIGs are the symbolic representations that have been internalized from peoples' early intersubjective experiences, their experiences of caregivers. For any individual, a RIG is a set of images, feelings, perceptions, and actions—a sort of *collage* of stimuli—that evokes the felt memories of significant caregiver interactions. Stern discusses the effects of RIGs on infants' sense of core relatedness, their ability to feel integrity and continuity in the presence of another. Let us look at Stern's example of the infant Stevie as an example of a RIG in action:

> Stevie experiences the following RIG: a high level of arousal, maternal behavior that tends to push him beyond his tolerable limits, the need to self-regulate downward, and the (usually) successful self-regulation by persistent aversions. . . . when he is experiencing the higher levels of excitement, his mother has become a different kind of evoked companion, a self-disregulating other. (p. 195)

Stern's "evoked companion" is a set of images and feelings that comes into being when a person experiences a RIG. The evoked companion is an accumulation of previously lived experiences rather than a representative of what is "out there." Even an adolescent or adult may impose such an evoked companion in a particular interpersonal situation that includes the stimuli of a RIG. (Obviously, a RIG is analogous to a parataxic distortion.) It is particularly the evocation of an intense emotional state that precipitates the organization of these RIGs. As Stern notes, some recent discoveries of the effect of mood on memory (e.g., Bower, 1981) seem to support the idea that intense affect organizes certain representational experiences.

Stern presents a brief clinical case of a 34-year-old man who has some similarity with Jerry. Stern uses information that he has gathered in the developmental history to explain current interpersonal problems:

> It was mainly with his wife that he felt not understood. He felt that instead of just listening to him she always became defensive, so that he was confronted by an adversary rather than an ally. Even in issues that involved no criticism, when he simply wanted to explain how he felt about something, she would too quickly jump in with unasked-for

suggestions about what to do. . . . When he wanted to be understood, he felt advised. (p. 268)

Additionally this man, who presented complaints about generalized depression and episodes of rage at his wife, experienced certain feelings of insecurity at work. He inhibited himself from taking risks, and he wanted to be taken under the wing of a senior colleague, although he loathed the fact that he wanted it. He felt dependent on his wife, but disliked this also. Stern interprets much of this behavior in regard to the evoked companions of an "intrusive other" with the wife, and a "protective other" with his seniors, as related to a significant depression in his mother during the formation of an intersubjective self, about 18 to 30 months of age.

The earliest period of the "emergent self" (0–3 months) is one in which temperament and environment (including the state of the infant's body) contribute to the formation of beginning subjectivity. Stern sees much evidence of individuality and a rudimentary integration of subjectivity during this very early state of self. The next period (3–9 months) Stern calls "core self," and it has to do especially with the establishment of an embodied sense of being and the recognition of others who are similarly coherent. Following directly is the period of "subjective self" (9–18 months), during which time the infant discovers and enacts a sense of "psychological being" or the experience of individual subjectivity. The final period, "verbal self," begins at about 18 months and continues on to contribute to all forms of communication and thought. These various self formations are formally without end points in that they are continuous and reworked through all experience. At any moment, a person has access to all of these states and may experience any one of them as primary. Each one is accompanied by certain kinds of interpersonal experience: emergent relatedness, core relatedness, intersubjective relatedness, and verbal relatedness. "Life-course . . . issues such as autonomy and attachment are worked on equally in all the domains of relatedness that are available at any given time" (Stern, p. 33).

To return to Stern's (1985) case of the 34-year-old man, we are told how the impact of his mother's depression might have influenced his intersubjective self and evoked companion in adulthood.

He experienced a painful rupture in intersubjective relatedness when his wife would not or could not enter into and share his subjective experience, so far as that is possible. It is likely that a heightened sensitivity to this form of interpersonal disjunction was established during the period when he was one to two and one-half years old. It is very likely that because of her depressive "preoccupations" his mother was relatively less available for intersubjective relatedness than for serving physically as a secure base of operations. (pp. 271–272)

Although we do not have early developmental information about Jerry, we could say that Jerry still had some obvious difficulties with subjective self at the time of beginning treatment. As Stern explains it, the various self formations are being reworked constantly at all phases of the lifespan. The interpersonal experience that accompanies the organization of the subjective self is that of intersubjective relating, the knowledge of other people as psychological individuals like oneself. Jerry has some difficulties with evoked companions, when he relates to women, and to men whom he admires. For example, Jerry's describes Cynthia as "having balls" and his envy of her independence gives us hints about what he might fear or avoid in contacts with women. On the other hand, Jerry is careful to treat admired men with respect and humility (e.g., his somewhat obsequious attitude toward Dr. Hall regarding fees and the demands of treatment) up to a point. That point is usually the one at which Jerry feels aggressive. The father who "wasn't there" emotionally is probably evoked when Jerry experiences himself as "too demanding" or "too impulsive." Jerry's first strategy is to seduce or flatter the evoked Father, and then his second strategy appears to be a version of "baring his throat" or showing his fear in a somewhat vulnerable or enfeebled way.

The RIGs (representations of interactions that have been generalized) that Jerry might experience in relation to the severity of both parents, but especially the direct and intrusive demands he experienced with his mother, probably push him into core-self difficulties. These are difficulties with the fundamental unity of being: coherence and continuity. Although we have no direct evidence from the case, it is likely that Jerry experiences himself as nonexistent from time to time, or at least as powerless. The implied sense of powerlessness is indicated both by Jerry's making hostile threats (as though he had no real power) and by Jerry's difficulties in identifying himself as a fully competent adult man.

The case gives us many examples of how Jerry's intersubjective relating with men evolved over the course of treatment. We are not privy to much information on the evolution in regard to women, however. The end of the report merely states that Jerry was able to tell his mother that he was living with his woman companion, although his mother disapproved. This single incident is not enough to determine whether or not Jerry has had adequate reworking of the RIGs involving his mother to be able to be empathically attuned to woman companions, and hence—to appreciate them on a fully intersubjective level.

Winnicott (1958, 1965, 1971) made many contributions to understanding subjectivity. As Greenberg and Mitchell (1983) say of Winnicott, "Almost all of his major contributions concerned the conditions making possible the child's awareness of himself as a being separate from other people . . ." (p. 191). As we mentioned earlier, for Winnicott it is the optimal failure of the "holding environment" (or good-enough mothering) that permits the development of psychological individuality. The ability to perceive another as an "object" (another subjectivity) rather than as an aspect of oneself is, according to Winnicott, "jogged along less effectually by satisfactions than by dissatisfactions. The satisfaction to be derived from a feed has less value in this respect. . . . Instinct-gratification gives the infant a personal experience and *does little to the position of the object . . .*" (Winnicott, 1965, p. 181, emphasis in original). Beginning in a fusion with caregivers, the infant gradually differentiates the self and other through frustrations. Optimal failure—whether through refusal on the part of a caregiver to cooperate with a demand or through circumstantial changes—becomes the basis of educating the infant to a not-me world, according to Winnicott. Adaptational failures have value according to the degree to which "the infant can hate the object" (p. 181)—to retain the idea that the caregiver is potentially satisfactory while recognizing the lack of satisfaction in the present moment. This ability to "destroy" the object (another person) in one's imagination, while recognizing that the object is not, in fact, destroyed is the basis of interpersonal trust.

Winnicott would also add that this kind of trust is a part of all communications that are truly "intersubjective," that belong to the world of psychological individuality. He says, "In so far as the object is subjective, *so far is it unnecessary for communication with it to be explicit*" (p. 182, emphasis in original). Once other people are experienced as coherent individuals, they are communicated to on a basis of explicit statements or nothing at all. Thus, with the recognition of the "objectivity" of the other, there appears both a new enjoyment of using specific modes of communication and the ability to isolate oneself or to stop communicating. Hence, one can recognize the "boundary" or coherence of self and other. There are no perceived threats then that another person can penetrate one's own subjectivity, nor any confusions about "reading" another's mind.

Emphasizing the necessity of both separation from, and vulnerability to, the other, Winnicott (1971) offers the example of "play" or the *potential space* between people as the optimal environment for self-development. He says, for example,

> In order to give a place to playing I postulated a *potential space* between the baby and the mother. . . . I contrast this potential space

(a) with the inner world (which is related to the psychosomatic partnership) and (b) with actual, or external, reality (which has its own dimensions, and which can be studied objectively, and which . . . does in fact remain constant). (1971, p. 41)

This potential space is the arena for the development of all intersubjective relating, hence all psychological individuality. Within this space, play is a central means by which early development takes place as well as the essence of effective psychotherapy (from Winnicott's point of view). Play is universally related to growth and health. When people are able to play they can use the external world to represent psychological realities *without* being confused about, or frightened by, this use. By manipulating external reality in the service of psychological meanings, a person is permitted to "try on" any number of possibilities both for his/her feeling expressions and ideas.

Furthermore, the capacity to play implies trust that the potential space can be used adaptively for one's needs. Playing is essentially satisfying or it is not playing at all. When anxiety or anger destroys the potential space, then playing reaches a saturation point at which the participants can no longer contain the experience within the metaphorical space. Winnicott assumed that psychotherapy was "done in the overlap of the two play areas, that of the patient and that of the therapist" (1971, p. 54). If the therapist cannot play, then the therapist is not suitable to the work, but if the patient cannot play, then the therapy must do something to enable the patient to develop this capacity because it is just this capacity that will foster the experience of differentiation that therapy is about.

Winnicott goes on to say that the "search for self" requires playing and the specific kind of creativity involved with play, this being different from the creativity involved in making works of art or other products. "It is in playing and only in playing that the individual child or adult is able to be creative and to use the whole personality, and it is only in being creative that the individual discovers the self" (1971, p. 54). All in all, Winnicott assumes that the experience of a sense of self requires relaxation under a condition of trust that is well-established, creative activity that is both physical and mental as manifested in play, and the reflecting back of these experiences from a valued other (p. 56).

In our case of Jerry, we can see that Jerry's capacity for play was limited by his anxiety at the beginning of treatment. Rather than being able to create and sustain a potential space with Dr. Hall, Jerry would occasionally disrupt the therapeutic space with actual threats or supplications and then say that he wanted to be "totally honest." Similarly, his assertion "I want to put my *penis* in you!"—made to the older, successful group member—is the kind of instinctual expression that specifically disrupts play. Jerry's difficulties with "trying to control the group" are yet another expression of his inability to relax and trust the creative aspects of the therapeutic situation.

Eventually, however, the group provided the right potential space for Jerry, and he began to play. Therapeutic failures in the holding environment of support for Jerry were optimal, from a Winnicott point of view. Although one man actually challenged Jerry to a fist fight (definitely *not* a playful affair and one that would "prove" the truly destructive nature of Jerry's aggression), he did not carry through. Dr. Hall's neutrality regarding the nature of group members' challenges to Jerry was a specific communication that their challenges were playful, metaphoric, not real threats.

Jerry's ability to accept his parents as "good enough" is a function of his new ability to accept Dr. Hall and the group members as trustworthy enough to play. As Winnicott (1971) says, "In these highly specialized conditions the individual can come together and exist as a unit, not as a defense against anxiety but as an expression of I AM, I am alive, I am myself" (p. 56). In a sense, the playfulness of Dr. Hall's comments about Jerry's workbench are an invitation to Jerry to experience his agency and coherence as "enough" to engage with others in a state of trust and reciprocity.

The three theorists we have reviewed in this section, Sullivan, Stern, and Winnicott, have taken some essentially different points of view on the nature of the self-system or the purpose of individual subjectivity. Sullivan avers that anxiety is the primary organizer of individuality and that the experience of self-separateness is essentially defensive and negative. The goal of development and personality is intimacy, and the self-system is the enemy of intimacy. Stern, on the other hand, assumes that individual subjectivity is already organized at birth. From his point of view it is biologically functional that the organism emerge immediately as an individual unit. Consequently it is not to be imagined that people begin their lives in a state of "fusion" or "symbiosis." These are dysfunctional by-products of problematic RIGs, emotional misattunements, and intrusive evoked companions.

From Stern's point of view, the experience of self is given in human life at birth. Our ability to develop it in relation to other subjectivities and then to maintain it optimally is contingent on our relationships, especially with our powerful caregivers of the first 3 years. From Winnicott's perspective, the experience of psychological individuality is contingent on a capacity to play. At birth we are fused or undifferentiated from those around us. It is a developmental achievement that the infant can experience the "object" (another person) as outside of itself. Only optimal failures of the facilitating environment permit the possibility for discriminating the boundaries of the self. Beyond the initial experiences of body–psyche collusion as a "separate" self, the capacity to experience the psychological nature of one's individuality depends on the potential space between people. That is, the experience of self depends on trust, relaxation, creativity, and reflections of all these from a trusted other. For Winnicott, then, the achievement of a truly psychological individuality is hard won and ongoing.

LICHTENBERG, LOEVINGER, AND KEGAN

Psychiatrist and psychoanalyst Lichtenberg (1989) has recently assembled a model of motivational–affective systems that characterizes both infant/child development and the major structures of adult personality functioning. Similar to Stern (1985), Lichtenberg stresses the role of subjectivity or self in the process of development. Lichtenberg offers a map for depicting "model scenes" from childhood that can be identified later in adulthood in metaphorical enactments of motivational functioning, especially in a therapeutic setting. Research psychologist Loevinger (Loevinger & Wessler, 1970; Loevinger, 1976) has gradually built a developmental model, derived empirically from 30 years of research using a sentence completion test. This model is a map of nine stages or frames of reference that depict different organizations of subjectivity, perhaps exhaustive of subjective organizations that people construct. Kegan (1982), a clinical–developmental psychologist who is also a researcher, has more recently assembled his own six stages of subjectivity—the evolving self—that are similar to Loevinger's, Kohlberg's (e.g., 1981), Gilligan's (1982), as well as others. His model is based, in part, on a clinical sample and attempts to take into account the relationship between development and psychiatric symptoms.

Lichtenberg departs from classical psychoanalytic theory in taking the self as a central concept. Here is his definition:

> Self refers to a center for initiating, organizing, and integrating. Sense of self refers to how initiating, organizing, and integrating are experienced. Sense of self as a container allows for a place to fit concepts such as agency, coherence of boundaries and locus for action, affective experience and continuity of sameness, the observed regularity of the flow of events. (1989, p. 57)

He goes on to say that *motivation* is the core of psychoanalytic theory and that he would like to integrate motivation with structure in his own approach. As Lichtenberg puts it, "The problem that has occupied me for the last several years is to define motivational systems that exist in early infancy, persist in altered forms throughout life, and characterize observable changes in motivational dominance in an analytic session" (p. 58).

Lichtenberg (1989) identifies five motivational–functional systems that are evident in neonates and adults: (1) fulfilling physiological requirements; (2) attachment and affiliation; (3) assertion and exploration; (4) aversive reactions of antagonism and withdrawal; and (5) sensual and sexual pleasure. Each one is connected with particular affective expressions, interpersonal patterns, and symbolic representations.

Similar to Stern, Lichtenberg especially stresses the developmental shift from a world of *interaction* to a world of *intersubjectivity*. Similar to Sullivan, Lichtenberg sees meeting physiological needs as a "rather quick-acting signal system conveying information of need and consummation to the caregiver and a feedback system conveying the same information to the emergent self" (p. 60). Needs have clear goals so that consummations can be easily matched by caregiver responses.

Tension, on the other hand, can easily disrupt the motivational system of attachment/affiliation—the tension of anxiety being a disintegrating tension in Lichtenberg's scheme as it was in Sullivan's. The motivational system of attachment/affiliation is enhanced through recurrent patterning of exchanges that involve consummation of physiological needs, but specific attachment needs can be met only through the emotional attunements of matching voice and movement so that the caregiver communicates tenderness.

From investigations of the chains and sequences of reciprocal behaviors that make up mother–infant interactions, Lichtenberg finds of central importance the caregiver's ability to follow and highlight, to elaborate and imitate, what the infant is expressing. It seems that the infant has the opportunity then for an experience of subjectivity, an organization of unity. In the first 18 months of life, infants respond to caregivers primarily in terms of two aspects of early subjectivity: affective experiences of shared arousal and intentional experiences of doing something together. The following statement is an example of how Lichtenberg understands this motivational system of attachment/ affiliation to continue to develop.

> The desire for affective attunement, for empathic resonance, for guidance as a relief from the distress of uncertainty, for the comfort of sharing intimacy, and for the sense of value that accrues from idealization is part of the structuring of the attachment motivational-

functioning system in infancy. These desires persist along with many wishes that develop as part of the complexity that comes with triangular attachments. (1989, p. 63)

The other motivational systems are similarly described from neonate behavior to adult functioning so that we can understand the textual themes of subjectivity that stretch from the beginning to the end of life.

Moreover, Lichtenberg regards each of these motivational systems as a sort of subpersonality with a biological and neurophysiological base to insure survival. Each system functions in a self-regulating capacity with its own hierarchy of organization from needs and learning schemas to perceptual–affective action patterns and symbolic representations. In speaking of his whole model of personality, Lichtenberg (1989) says,

I regard *needs* as fundamental requirements for biological survival and psychic integrity, and I regard wishes as an infinite variety of conscious and unconscious motives that derive from needs in the course of development. When a need in any of the motivational–functional systems is met, an emotional value is added. (p. 68)

When needs and wishes are relatively compatible, then a person experiences a basically congruent and harmonious interplay of these motivational systems in the overall unity of self-regulation. When needs and wishes are persistently in conflict or uncoordinated, then patterns or structures of a pathological nature develop. From the point of view of *needs*, the pathological patterns represent deficits in self-regulation of one or more motivational systems. Looked at from the point of view of conflicting *wishes*, the patterns represent intrapsychic conflicts that pit motivations against each other.

In a clinical situation, as in the case of Jerry, the therapist can read the affective–motivational patterns and look for indications of "model scenes"—both prototypical and paradigmatic for action–affect organization. Model scenes are similar to RIGs and evoked companions in that they introduce into the current moment certain feelings, images, desires, and actions that are aspects of earlier subjectivity. In order to become an expert with a particular client's model scenes, the therapist has to call on the transferential field and her/his own experiences of the moment. In the case of Jerry, we have only the written report, but we can capture some of the dynamic interplay in terms of his early repeated actions with the close women in his life, members of the group, and Dr. Hall.

Let us take the motivational system of aversive reactions of antagonism and withdrawal. Aversive reactions undergo the same hierarchy of transformation developmentally: from innate, to learned, to planned, to symbolically represented. Aversive responses are optimally used to deal with conflict and negotiation, as expressions of anger. At times they become subsumed under a self-protective or self-preservative function of aggression. Parents provide protection for the infant and child so that the aversive system can be responsive to what is required, safe, and acceptable behavior. Feelings of shame, embarrassment, and guilt are induced by parents and draw into conflict certain need motivations with specific wishes and values, such as "Don't bite or hit other people."

Clearly Jerry's aversive motivational system activates some kind of model scene when he verbalizes threats to Dr. Hall or to the group members, when he is unable to empathize with his withdrawing woman friend, and when he is fearful that larger corporations will oust him. It is very likely that Jerry's aversive needs are in conflict with his wishes and that his wishes carry few value-laden organizations. Jerry seems to enact a sort of "identification with the aggressor" when he makes challenging, aggressive statements that are otherwise out of context. Typically this kind of primitive motivational system is an expression of repeated traumatic experiences in childhood or infancy. It is as if this particular system exists somehow outside of the realm of Jerry's ordinary sense of himself. It is something like a "not-me" experience both when it "happens" to Jerry and as it is communicated to others. The case report does not clarify whether Jerry came to symbolize or to plan his aversive responses as a result of therapeutic interventions. We should assume some improvement in this direction because the group members gradually came to accept and even respect him.

In shifting our analysis to Loevinger's theory, we move away from the implications of reconstructing the past in the present. Ego development is a model, derived from research using sentence completion tests, that is substantially different from most of the other models we have used here because (1) it is not clinically derived and (2) it is not predicated on particular events in childhood or infancy, hypothesized or observed. Loevinger (Loevinger & Wessler, 1970; Loevinger, 1976) and her colleagues have worked over the last 30 years to standardize a scoring procedure for a projective measure that uses open-ended sentence stems (e.g., The thing I like about myself . . .) to characterize different types or patterns of subjectivity.

The model that has developed from these empirical investigations of thousands of people consists of nine stages or frames of reference. Ego development theory is based on constructivist (e.g., Piaget and Kelly) models as well as on psychoanalytic (e.g., Freud and Sullivan) concepts. It has become a useful assessment tool in the hands of clinical–developmental psychologists who want to understand the relationship between types of subjectivity and types of therapeutic interventions.

As we said above, it is possible that the ego development model is exhaustive of the types or patterns of subjective organization that persons construct. Although Loevinger uses the term "ego" rather than "self," she defines her ego differently from the structural model of Freudian psychoanalysis. Loevinger's (1976) ego is a relatively well-organized frame of reference a person brings to experience, the lens through which the data of experience are perceived and arranged into unities of "self" and "other."

In the context of ego development, we can assume that the self or ego is restricted to the *organization* of perceptions, feelings, and beliefs about individual subjectivity (and other subjectivities) that allows a person to go on being a self-recognized unity. As we said above, from the research of Lewis et al. (1989), self-recognition and self-conscious emotions begin roughly in the second half of the second year of life. This is apparently the beginning of individual construction of self, but Loevinger's method of research—depending as it does on the ability to read and write and respond with concentration to a written test—is valid only after about the age of 11 or 12. The data on which the Loevinger model is based are, therefore, from adolescents and adults.

The nine stages described by Loevinger begin with a *presocial stage* that is prior to her empirical investigation. This stage is one in which language cannot be used to organize and represent experiences. Obviously people who remain in this stage even through childhood are unable to function without custodial care. The next stage is called *impulsive* and involves the organization of a primarily body-based self to monitor and control certain basic impulses. Adults at this stage are barely able to function without supervision; they are not able to assume full adult responsibility; their sentence completions are impoverished (e.g., okay, nice, good, pissed), and they react rather than respond to the instrument. Following the impulsive stage is the *self-protective stage* in which the focus is on fears, troubles, and wishes. Adults at this stage may be complex and intelligent, although they are primarily motivated to protect their own interests and manipulate situations to increase pleasure and avoid trouble.

The *conformist stage*, which follows, is one in which identification with the "group" and obedience to rules are predominant. A desire to belong and be approved of is central and tends to motivate people to overcome self-protective fears and schemes in favor of the group's good. Girl Scout/Boy Scout morality pervades, and stereotypes and clichés abound at this stage. Next comes the *self-aware stage* in which a person is awakened to a diversity of norms and values as legitimate. Although stereotyping and dualistic thinking continue, a person at this stage begins to recognize that "differences" are inherent in the human condition, although these are understood as "the way people are" (are born, usually) rather than as connected to context. Personal meanings are perceived in more complex ways than at earlier stages. Right–wrong, good–bad, even self–other are no longer discrete and reliable categories. Because this person has no coherently established personal identity, and because the person still externalizes authority, she/he feels acute pressure to "find myself."

At the next stage, the *conscientious stage*, there clearly emerges for the first time an awareness that the past and future relate to the present and hence that "psychological development" is possible. Diversity of norms and values is accepted and understood as related to context. Personal achievement and relational responsibility are the affectively charged themes, themes that may provoke a true identity crisis when they are in conflict with each other. Formal operational thought can be applied to a range of experience, including oneself and one's thoughts and feelings. Mutuality and cooperation are conscious ideals for interpersonal relating, and the conflict between the group and the individual is no longer seen as problematic. Rather, this kind of conflict is expected, and conventional goals are somewhat shunned. Guilt and perfectionism complicate the picture of a subjectivity that is hedged around with self-imposed demands to be one's "brother's keeper" and one's own fountain of wisdom.

At the *individualistic stage* these desires for perfection are partly supplanted by the desire for self-fulfillment. Conflicts continue, however, between autonomous pursuits, for example, work or studies, and relational responsibility. As the title suggests there is a strong emphasis on individuality at this stage and concern about existential issues and conflicts. The other postconscientious stages, *autonomous* and *integrated*, include a fuller sense of personal identity, the acceptance of conflict as a part of human life, and a greater tolerance for ambiguity and paradox.

These nine organizations of subjectivity are somewhat correlated with chronological development, up to a point. That point appears to be the self-aware stage. From a variety of studies it appears that the self-aware stage is the modal stage for adults in North America. The ego development scheme can thus be considered to be both a developmental hierarchy or continuum of stages and a typology of different subjectivities among adults. We take it to be an account of the different theories or constructs of self/other that adults bring to experience.

This model is not intended to be a model of adaptation or mental health in which "higher is better." Considering the model to be a presentation of self/other configurations, we explicitly exclude the chaotic disorganization of types of pathology. These are by definition "not self" or are "outside" of the organization. Events such as fragmentation of self-coherence, disruptions of intentionality, disturbances of continuity, and nonaccess to emotional arousal can and do occur at *all* stages. Responses to such impingements appear to differ by stages, however.

Jerry is a case in point. Although Jerry has difficulty containing his impulses to attack others, he does not actually attack them. Jerry puts his desire into words, saying "I want to" do something aggressive. The manner in which Jerry handles disruptive anxiety and the goals and desires he sets for himself depict a *self-aware stage* of ego development. For example, Jerry consciously wants to "create the impression" that he has a larger staff and office. He has doubts about his ability to have an independent consulting job, but he is also afraid of "sudden dismissal" if he works for a corporation. Jerry's solicitousness and his desire to be approved of by Dr. Hall and the group members, as well as his confusion about how to belong to the group, are all indicators of self-aware functioning. Jerry seems to be confused about how to follow rules without making them dictates, and he desires direct advice and support, although he can clearly do without it (as, for example, his ability to deal with Dr. Hall's neutral approach).

The ego development model permits the therapist to answer questions about treatment with greater confidence. For instance, the self-aware stage is especially well suited to group psychotherapy because the focal conflict at this stage is the relationship of individual to group, the understanding of individual differences. Additionally, people at this stage are capable of insight and benefit from insight-oriented therapies, especially from those involving aspects of conformity to a group, such as family therapy or group therapy.

The individual therapeutic relationship with a client at the self-aware stage is often more difficult than those with clients at later (and even earlier) stages. Ambivalent and skeptical about authority, the self-aware client will test the therapist's expertise and validity in a way reminiscent of a teenager's testing of parental advice. Often the client has "suspicions" that she/he knows more than the therapist does "about life." The client may find it difficult to endorse the therapist's authority, but she/he will be very disappointed if the therapist does not assume a position of authority and confidence. Status and qualifications (recall that Jerry heard Dr. Hall in a public lecture and knew he was an "analyst") of the therapist are more important at this stage than at earlier, and even later, ones.

Obviously Jerry eventually responded to the parameters of group treatment (where he was a member and not a leader), and individual treatment where he was expected to take responsibility for interpreting his dreams and understanding his own associations. Jerry seems to be moving toward the conscientious stage in which there is a greater sense of responsibility for one's part in relationships and a greater ability to "play" with the metaphors of psychological life.

Although Kegan's (1982) model of stage development has many similarities to Loevinger's, it also has some differences. From the beginning of his work, Kegan has been interested in developmental psychopathology, especially in understanding the relationship between the process of differentiation/integration and pathological dysfunction.

In a recent paper, Rogers and Kegan (1989) remark that most theories of developmental psychopathology attempt to account for adolescent and adult difficulties in terms of early dysfunctions or patterns of relationship. These theories, in predicting pathology based on early life, necessarily overlook the significance of self-reflection, formal operational thought, and other complexities of later cognitive development. In order to study the possible relationships between forms of adult and adolescent development and experiences of psychopathology, Rogers and Kegan focus on "deep structures" or the "orthogenetic principle" of Werner (1957). This is the idea that development proceeds always from a state of less to greater differentiation, articulation, and hierarchic integration.

In general, they have not found a clear positive relationship between the severity of psychological disturbance and the stage of cognitive–structural development. Instead, they have found a significant relationship between the *form* of disturbance and the stage of development. Disturbances that involve actions and impulses (in which emotional responses are acted out rather than symbolically represented) correlate with lower stages of development in their findings. Disturbances of thought, involving even psychotic thought processes, that are expressed through symbolic representation, correlate with higher stages of development.

Rogers and Kegan (1989) claim that the biological model of growth dominates current thinking about development and psychopathology. Therefore, many theorists of developmental psychopathology believe that the earliest stages of human development are the most flexible and vulnerable. According to this principle, a very disruptive psychological symptom (such as fragmentation of the self) would have its roots in early traumas or distresses.

Rogers and Kegan emphasize a different principle of psychological development. They say,

> Perhaps a better way of conceptualizing personality structure would be in terms of the underlying motive of the self to organize experience into a coherent whole. . . . We would then be able to describe how

late-occurring disruptions to the stability of that coherence may affect
all or many aspects of organized experience. (p. 13)

The self-reflective thought of later development and more mature processes of representation and judgment are the focus of Kegan's concern.

Basically two studies have been conducted to test the hypothesis
that types of psychopathology are related to developmental functioning:
the first one, reported in Kegan (1982), involved 45 adolescent and adult
inpatients on an acute psychiatric unit, ranging in age from 16 to 70.
Researchers employed Kohlberg's (Colby & Kohlberg, 1987) methodolo-
gy of the moral dilemma interview, and the symptom lists of severity
developed by Zigler and Phillips (Zigler & Glick, 1986) to investigate
the hypothesized relationship. They found that more "immediate, be-
haviorally expressed symptoms such as impulsive and aggressive actions" correspond to earlier stages of moral development and that "more
mediated symptoms of ideational disturbances expressed in delusional
thinking and self-depreciation" correspond with later stages of moral
development (Rogers & Kegan, 1989, p. 30).

In the second study, two independent sources of structural development were used: the moral dilemma interview and an experience-based
interview that was coded using an adapted version of Selman's (1980)
conceptions of self/other. The second, more clinical interview permitted
the investigators to look closely at the relationship between self-
reflective thought and psychiatric symptoms. The study participants
were 41 adolescent and young adult patients on an inpatient acute
psychiatric unit, ranging in age from 16 to 25. They were interviewed
three times each and were asked to complete a number of self-report
measures relevant to their psychiatric symptoms. Again they found
support for the idea that symptom expression changes with development.
They found

> a shift in the form of psychiatric symptom expression from overt,
> impulsive actions and demands where frustration is expressed di-
> rectly and through action . . . to disturbances of subjective thought
> processes, doubt, and self-recrimination, and flight from accepted
> social realities. . . . (p. 34)

Within all diagnostic grouping of symptoms, the form of the symptom
was related to the developmental status of the patient. For example,
within the group of patients whose primary diagnosis was psychosis
(acute psychosis, schizophrenia, schizoaffective disorder), there was a
range of symptoms expressed from both action and thought categories;
this range varied with developmental status.

From earlier studies and other models of stage development, Kegan (1982) assembled his model of the "evolving self." His model presents six stages that are quite similar in their interpersonal themes to Loevinger's stages: *incorporative, impulsive, imperial, interpersonal, institutional,* and *interindividual.* (The title "institutional" is less explanatory than the others; it refers to identity and self-authorship, typically involving career, role, and public arenas; this corresponds to "conscientious" in Loevinger's model.) For each stage Kegan presents complex descriptions that range from descriptions of "subject–object differentiation" and "holding environment" (context) to functions of "confirming, contradicting, continuing," and leaving a stage.

We can take as an example the *interpersonal stage,* which generally characterizes Jerry's development. The differentiation of subjectivity is expressed in terms of inner states, mutuality of feelings, particular feelings, and personal values and ideals. The differentiation of objectivity is expressed in terms of enduring dispositions in others, others' needs and interests, and the actuality of others' being. Although Jerry seems to fit the subjective description, he may fall short of being able to discriminate enduring needs and qualities in others. His recent involvement with his neighbors and his ability to admire certain stable qualities in them may be an expression of a new ability. Certainly at the beginning of treatment he acted as though others existed only in his fantasy, through his own egocentric perceptions, and for his own uses.

The "holding environment" for the interpersonal stage is a mutually reciprocal one-to-one relationship, originally called a "chum" by Sullivan. The dynamic orientation of this stage is expressed in many of Jerry's newfound friendships: they involve sharing feelings, assuming responsibility for one's own intiatives, and recognizing the reality of "other people." The medium of transition out of this stage and into the next, the institutional stage, is some kind of "provisional identity." Going away to college or the military might typically provide the bridge into the next stage of development, but in Jerry's case the provisional identities of divorce and "being a consultant" may have the same effect. Additionally, being a member of a psychotherapy group gives one an opportunity to "try on" a new identity with the full knowledge that one will move on to something else soon.

Both Loevinger's and Kegan's stage models provide lenses through which we can see Jerry in his current functioning. These viewpoints allow us to understand more about motivating new development and intervening to assist him in maintaining his current level under stress.

There is a contrast between these last two constructivist models and the other models that tended to assume the repetition of the past in the present character of subjectivity. Loevinger and Kegan simply characterize present subjectivity without reasoning about a past. Neither Loevinger nor Kegan is ready to explain why some people "go on" developing in adulthood and others do not. Principally it appears that we need more study of the relationship between adolescent/adult knowledge structures and the symptoms of psychological disturbance in order to understand structural change in adults.

This chapter has presented a full round of lenses through which to view Jerry's subjectivity. Our goal has been to motivate our readers to understand configurations of self from different theoretical models, each one lending new meanings to understanding the characteristics of stability and change of self. Our wide-ranging tour through self theories also provides the possibility now of comparing Jung's model with other contemporary models. In the next chapter, we present a Jungian analysis of Jerry and some of the interpretations provided by Dr. Hall regarding his understanding of this fragment of a case.

☆ 8 ☆

The Case of
Jerry from
a Jungian Perspective

A Jungian approach to understanding Jerry opens the way now to compare Jung's self psychology with the other 12 models we applied in the previous chapter. In the final chapter we make explicit comparisons between Jung and other self theorists. In this chapter, we intend to show the manner in which we, as Jungian analysts and constructivists, would work with Jerry, and the way in which Jung's ideas illuminate the clinical material.

Our constructivist orientation toward Jung's theory means that we embrace only the aspects of the theory that link to a clear sense of the psychological construction of the world. For example, we use the idea of *archetype* as a predisposition to form a coherent image in an emotionally aroused state. We consider all psychological complexes to have cohered around archetypal images of core emotional arousal. Practically speaking, this eliminates the distinction between the "personal" unconscious organized by complexes and the "collective" unconscious organized by archetype. Each psychological complex is both personal and collective. The association of personal images, ideas, and actions (i.e., semantic and episodic memories) around a core arousal state connected with an archetypal image is the basic organizing structure for *all* of personality in this use of Jungian theory.

In the case of Jerry, for instance, the father complex is organized around an image of a destructive, overwhelming, negative father. This archetypal motif—represented universally in images of demon, devil, evil, and attacking men—is connected with emotional states of fear/

138

aggression and anger. These are universal or collective aspects of human affective experience, but the personal aspects of Jerry's own complex connect with feelings and enactments of abandonment, criticism, belittlement, and resentment that are the particular products of *his* experiences of a demanding, judgmental, potentially cruel, and controlling father to whom Jerry believed he had to submit.

Both of us (Young-Eisendrath, 1984, 1985; Young-Eisendrath & Wiedemann, 1987; Hall, 1977, 1989) have written extensively on the clinical uses of the Jungian theory of psychological complexes. To clarify various aspects of our application of Jungian theory to this case, we quote from our earlier work. Hall (1989) emphasizes the interaction of personal and archetypal themes in parental complexes:

> Experiences with the personal parents are as likely to limit the archetypal potentialities of the child's psyche as they are to enhance them. All children have the capacity to be loving and affectionate, but that innate ability can be severely diminished and distorted if they are unable to actualize it easily with a parent of sufficient maturity and stability. It appears that the complexes underlying consciousness are comprised of collections of such experiences of interaction, thus providing both an ego-pole and an other-pole within the same structure of complexes. (p. 30)

Hall stresses also that psychological complexes are organized in aroused states of emotion, and those that are the concern of psychotherapy are frequently states of negative emotion. Psychological complexes treated in psychotherapy usually appear to relate to failures of parents (or, by extension, the environment that should support parenting, e.g., economic resources) to provide a sufficiently coherent and continuous environment so that archetypal potentials can develop and a child can mature from infancy to early adulthood.

Young-Eisendrath and Wiedemann (1987) stress the intersubjective nature of psychological complexes as they are experienced in relationships, and especially in the therapeutic relationship:

> A complex in interpersonal relating is experienced as a habitual field of action, symbol, and emotion organized around a core state of emotional arousal. . . . An unconscious complex may be projected onto someone else, or it may be momentarily identified with and taken on as an alien attitude. When an unconscious complex overtakes one's conscious identity, the person feels "beside herself" with strange moods, anxieties, and ideas. (p. 37)

In therapy and in other relationships, when alien complexes are discharged, people feel afraid and beside themselves. Complexes frequently create barriers to authentic relationships as old patterns and images are re-enacted and experienced as if they were absolute and timeless.

Hall (1989) stresses that it is possible for a rather severe unconscious complex to "remain dormant unless constellated by inner or outer events" and that such a complex may be discerned in projective testing (as Jung discovered in his use of word-association testing), in creative expressions (such as expressive arts), and in dreams but may remain unknown to the person (p. 33). Most therapeutic interventions cultivate the expression of psychological complexes in the second stage of therapy (the first stage involving the securing of rapport or therapeutic alliance). The third stage of therapy then promotes greater understanding and control of the enactment of complexes through rational (e.g., interpretation) or nonrational (e.g., creative practices) means.

When a person first comes for analytic treatment, the complexes structuring the personality are already in place. The therapist begins to map or assess them from the characteristics of the interactive field (therapist's experiences of the relationship with client) and from dreams, projective testing, creative activities, and/or the reported life story. Complexes never completely disappear—that is, they cannot be "analyzed away"—because they actually form the basis for continuity and coherence—for stability—in the personality. As a person changes, however, the arrangement and centrality of complexes change. Moreover, in therapy, a person comes to know and understand the symbolic meaning connected to complexes and can therefore establish an intrapsychic relationship to them, a relationship to one's own entrenched scripts, dramas, or habits of mind.

Emotion—in its expression and evocation—is the basis for the "constellation" or appearance of an individual's complexes. As Hall (1989) says

> Complexes form as the residue of all experiences. They are continually being formed and dissolved—*coagulat et solve*—just as the mineral content of bones is being continually dissolved and replaced. Usually complexes form slowly over long periods of time, but they may also be seen to form rapidly in situations of strong affect that threaten to overwhelm the self . . . (p. 33)

As we explained earlier, the archetype of the self is the core of its own psychological complex—the ego complex (sometimes called "self-images" in the following discussion)—that is aroused especially in relation to self-conscious emotions (pride, shame, envy, guilt, embarrassment) self-recognition, and self-reflection. In waking life we strive to organize our experiences of agency, coherence, continuity, and arousal according to the images, ideas, and actions of this identity complex. Obviously, though, from moment to moment we may identify with a non-self complex—such as a parental complex—and act and sound like someone else.

Jungian theory stresses the dissociative nature of personality. No complex entirely controls the personality, nor should it, although the ego complex is usually dominant during waking life. When a person entirely identifies with the ego complex, however, generally a neurosis develops as other complexes are repressed and denied. Identification with another complex (not-ego, not-I) is a dissociative state that may be severe (such as in multiple-personality disorder or psychotic states) or transient and temporary (such as in a mood).

As we said in Chapter 5, dreaming and the transcendent function are the means by which the conscious personality is corrected or balanced by the influence of other complexes; strong defenses against these influences lead to a one-sided overly rational, repressive, and controlling personality that is the prototype of Kohut's (1984) "guilty man." Kohut's other prototype, "tragic man," is the personality in which parental standards or values (e.g., conscience and restraint) are not integrated. Tragically, such a person is unable to stop identifying with being a child. Self-pity and envy, as we said earlier, are prominent aspects of this second condition, often categorized as a "personality disorder." Self-pity and envy are aspects of Jerry's inability to "grow up," also witnessed in his projections of the father complex onto authoritative males around him, while he identifies himself as the youthful, vulnerable son.

Before we assess Jerry more completely, a brief word about working with the transferential field in Jungian analysis (from a constructivist point of view). The interpersonal field is always potentially "charged" with complexes projected or identified with. In any relationship, but especially in affective relationships (such as parenting, therapy, or marriage), certain cues and/or ideas or actions may stimulate the constellation of a psychological complex. In this moment of affective arousal, the complex takes on a life of its own, as it were. If the complex is a difficult, dissociated one, or is an alien complex, it is likely to have a more shocking effect; it is less well known to the person.

Jung (CW 16) presents his understanding of the transferential field in alchemical terms with images of coagulation and solution that fit his experiences of psychological complexes. Contemporary Jungian analyst William Goodheart (1980) has offered a more interpersonal understanding of the phases of transferential/contertransferential dynamics in a Jungian analysis. Goodheart calls the first phase "persona-restoring" and notes that both analyst and analysand return to their "professional appearances" very predictably. The analyst is the well-behaved "good therapist," and the analysand is the similarly well-behaved "good client." At this point the two people *are* easily experienced as two distinct, separate people. At some point, however, when the analysand is trusting enough to feel something *authentic* in regard to the analyst, the analysand is likely to expect something from the analyst. With this shift, there is a gradual and (usually) irregular emergence of the second phase of the treatment, the "complex-discharging" phase when the analyst and analysand "mix together." During this phase (which comes and goes throughout a treatment), the analysand (especially) enacts psychological complexes (both troubling and ideal) within the therapeutic relationship. These enactments may involve projection and/or identification. They may be characterized as happening "out there" (in regard to wife, husband, or boss), or experienced as arising from material "in here" within the therapy.

To complicate matters further, the analyst's complexes may also be triggered as the analysand's parental complexes (especially idealizing and aggressive/sadistic) are projected. Pride, shame, envy, and guilt are frequently encountered in this phase on the part of both therapeutic partners as they struggle to reconstitute an ordinary sense of self within the analytic treatment. The analyst's ability to withstand negative and idealized transferences while maintaining the therapeutic alliance (the "kinship libido" in Jung's language) is the nitty-gritty of this second phase. Eventually, as the analysand is able to trust the interpretations discovered in the course of the treatment, the analysand is able progressively to claim the meaning and purpose of the psychological complexes enacted.

Analysand and analyst together develop a relationship to the complexes and share a symbolic attitude toward the material arising in the therapy. This is the initiation of the third phase, that of "symbol securing." The symbol-securing therapeutic field comes and goes in the final phase of a treatment. It is not always available because primitive complexes may be discharged even (and especially) during the termination phase of treatment. During symbol-securing, the analysand and analyst are once again two distinct people, this time with a sense of understanding the complexes (both genetically and finalistically) that arise in the field. Dreams, transferential cues, countertransferential cues, and reports of daily life all serve as evidence for the meaning and purpose of the complexes enacted and represented.

By the end of a Jungian treatment, the analysand and the analyst both will have changed. There is a progressive integration of the affect-laden meaning systems that are embodied in both of them. Psychological complexes of self and other form the basic structures of human personality universally and provide the basis for all of culture. Analysis allows us to talk about them and their images in a way that provides greater conscious awareness and sometimes greater control.

ASSESSMENT OF THE PROBLEM AND PERSONALITY

Jerry is in some ways a "classic Jungian case" because he is in midlife and he is searching for new ways to understand himself. He chose Dr. Hall because Dr. Hall aroused emotion, albeit a somewhat negative emotion. Jerry was "game" for authentic treatment and did not want merely to be supported or advised by a friendly therapist. Jerry's problem, from a Jungian perspective, is a powerful "puer complex." A classic Jungian description of this syndrome is *Puer Aeternus: A Psychological Study of the Adult Struggle with the Paradise of Childhood* by Marie-Louise von Franz (1981). Although Jerry did not appear to have had a paradisial childhood, it is his failure to depart from the fantasy or wish to be perfectly met, protected, and sustained that qualifies him for this classification.

The term *puer aeternus* is Latin for "eternal boy" (the feminine form is *puella aeternus*). The most widely accepted Jungian interpretation of this syndrome is von Franz's; von Franz sees it as a difficulty in detaching from the positive mother complex. The beloved son of the Great Mother (e.g., Eros of Venus) or the abandoned son of the Terrible Mother (e.g., Oedipus of Jocasta) are archetypal images of conditions in which it is difficult for the son to detach his identity from the positive mother complex and become a man (a father) himself. Instead, such a son feels a sense of entitlement that makes ordinary work (for advancement, for example, or material support) seem unappealing or even repugnant. It seems to the son that the positive mother complex (projected onto the actual mother, certain women, the world, or the analyst) should *confer* the desired result rather than having to earn it. A man dominated by a puer complex tends to live a "provisional life," living *as if* he were always preparing for life rather than doing it. Such a person is always *waiting* to receive the attention or reward that *provides* for him in proportion to his feelings of importance. (These feelings compensate for his fears of abandonment and emptiness, or his sense of worthlessness.)

In terms of Jerry's actual complexes, he presents himself as looking much younger than his age and avoids working for a large corporation because he fears dependence on it. His persona displays a *puer* quality when he treats authoritative men as if they should be submitted to or accept his "playful" or "pretend" threats. (Dr. Hall has remarked that he believes that Jerry's appearance and manner have probably changed little since his late adolescence; Jerry is now 49 years old.) Frequently, over the course of treatment, Jerry would speak about his desire to be admired for his appearance, even to the extent (communication from Dr. Hall, not in the case presentation) that he asked a homosexual man in the group to tell him whether he found him (Jerry) to be sexually attractive—although he (Jerry) was supposedly terrified of being thought to be homosexual! The desire to be admired had overtaken even his obsessive fears at that moment.

Often a person suffering from a *puer* complex has a father complex that is severe, demanding, critical, rejecting, or abandoning. Jerry is, of course, no exception. The negative father complex essentially "supports" or "sustains" the puer/mother alliance. This father complex carries the negative *senex* or "nasty old man" as a split-off, dissociated aspect of Jerry. Identifying himself with being youthful, promising, attractive, and sensitive/vulnerable, Jerry can imagine that other "older" men are aggressive, severe, demanding, critical, and/or emotionally empty or rigid. Other men can be imagined to be negative fathers (the "dominating and driven" patriarchs we read about) or to be positive mother–fathers (accepting, supporting, sustaining, and loving). As long as he imagines other men to have these qualities, then he must obey their commands, either to avoid their punishments or to seek their protection. Jerry's polite and empathic approach to Dr. Hall is symptomatic of this orientation. Similar, however, are some of his desires to help others who suffer, even to be "junior therapist" in doing so. Both desirable and undesirable aspects are evident in Jerry's persona.

Jerry's *shadow* complex is essentially the negative father. His persona covers the underlying rage, demand, and entitlement that emerge quickly when Jerry is vying for power. Frequently in the puer, one sees the negative father complex as the shadow that is both projected and intermittently identified with. For instance, Jerry's friends and family know about his demands, rage, and entitlement, but it is likely that Jerry dissociates these from his persona. He probably sees himself as a "nice guy."

Jerry's *anima* complex has been split between the sustaining good mother and the powerful negative mother. The good mother is imagined to be more accessible through men than women, it seems. This is possibly because Jerry perceived his own mother as overwhelming, frightening, and demanding. Jerry has criticized Dr. Hall (his positive mother–father) for not giving "enough" (communication from Dr. Hall) throughout the treatment. Jerry has always criticized his mother for giving in entirely the wrong ways or not at all. He imagines his women friends to be resourceful, powerful, competent, and frequently ungiving or giving in the wrong ways. If his women friends do not cater to his needs, they may provoke his rage and enactments of the negative father, along with the contention that *they* (the women) "made me so mad."

Overall, the puer complex has been assimilated into a developing ego complex (rather than the ego complex having assimilated to the puer). This means that Jerry has certain subjective strengths that he can count on and that permit him to function over a range of adult activities without depleting his self-esteem. For example, Jerry has been an agent in his own life. He has a successful consulting business, supports his teenage daughters, and has acted responsibly in regard to his ex-wife. Jerry has not abused drugs or alcohol. He can usually rely on self-reflection when he gets into a complex, even the more primitive aspects of self-pity, envy, and rage.

For these reasons, we would see Jerry as being delayed and hampered in his capacity for full adult functioning (family/relationship, work, and purpose) but not entirely thwarted. Jerry does not have a "personality disorder" of puer complex, but rather a problematic well-defended puer complex that sometimes dominates his personality. When? Mostly when he is "perceiving" others as though they were his parents: projecting the dominating negative mother complex onto women, or projecting the critical, abandoning father complex onto men. (Note: the projection of the anima—in this case the positive or negative mother—is an occasion of self–self/object interaction that is imbued with issues related to love.) By our assessment, then, the fundamental capacity for self-awareness is regularly available to Jerry. Jerry is capable of functioning effectively in a psychotherapy group and of integrating the reflections of others. Moreover, the opportunities afforded by the group (to understand his shadow and its projection, for instance) are critical to Jerry because his persona is very well-defended. Group members have confronted Jerry's persona and revealed its implied meanings, from subservience to superiority. Jerry has been able gradually to integrate these confrontations and to change.

COURSE OF TREATMENT, DREAMS, AND TRANSFERENTIAL FIELD

Before we talk specifically about Jerry's treatment, we want to make some general comments about Jungian analysis and psychotherapy. In contrast to most other analytical approaches, Jungian treatment spans a wide range of possible methods and means. Jungian analysts are themselves trained to use Freudian (often including object relations) approaches, Adlerian methods, Jungian methods, and sometimes other approaches. Depending on the training institute, a Jungian analyst may have actually completed a Freudian and/or Kleinian analysis in addition to a Jungian analysis. Whatever the training institute, all training candidates complete at least seminar training in other modes of analysis— Freudian psychoanalysis always, and, these days, usually the self psychology of Kohut, and often some other object relations approaches.

Jung was the first advocate for "matching" psychotherapeutic approaches to the personality of the client. Rather than matching the approach to the symptom, Jung believed that the personality of the client should be the determining factor along with the chronological age and/or place in the lifespan (for example, if a young person were dying, that person would be treated as being in the final phase of life). Jung assumed (see Ellenberger, 1970, for instance) that some "types" (using his typology, for example, the "extraverted thinking" type) would respond best to Freudian psychoanalysis. Other types (e.g., extraverted sensation and even feeling types) might respond better to an Adlerian approach. Still other types (for example, extraverted and introverted intuitives) would benefit most from Jungian treatment. He tended to base his judgment more on inferences about types of personality and types of psychotherapy than on a full understanding of the transferential field.

Whatever the theoretical approach, and whether or not the analyst uses the couch and/or a more "neutral" or "abstinent" style or uses face-to-face chairs with a more emotionally expressive style, Jungian analysts are trained to cultivate a therapeutic alliance. Jung stressed the necessity of a "real relationship" or the kinship bond in analysis. In this basic rapport with the analysand (founded on the belief that archetypal reality is universal, and universally a struggle), the analyst is clearly a colleague, a partner, and a collaborator. The activity and evidence of collaboration may not clearly emerge until the third phase of the treatment, however. An attitude of modesty and collaboration must be implicit in the analyst from the start, however.

For that reason, Jung advocates a certain kind of humility, an attitude of discovery with each new treatment. Rather than approaching the treatment with the idea that one already knows how to proceed, one approaches with the idea that one will discover how to proceed. This is "informed discovery" (see Young-Eisendrath, 1984) and not pure mystery. The analyst comes prepared with self-awareness, a knowledge of development, a variety of therapeutic methods, an ability to map complexes, and an attitude of interest or inquiry. Moreover, a Jungian analyst has a broad and fairly developed understanding of the human lifespan with a deep respect for the transitional events that mark each of the passages from infancy to old age. This means that the analyst believes that certain things "should be happening" in the course of a human lifetime. Again, this is not a strong formulaic dogma but rather a sense that human life is constrained by individuation and embodiment for all of us. Only the narcissistic identification with the ego and/or persona predisposes a person to ignore the passage of time and the meaning of human rites and rituals that signal maturity and decline.

Beyond these overarching themes, Jungian analysts vary greatly in how they specifically proceed with treatment methods. The three phases of treatment (described above) are always attended, and dream interpretation is almost always used (because it is considered a great resource for understanding compensation). Other methods may include on-the-couch "abstinent" analysis, on-the-couch more engaged (facing client) analysis, sandtray (creative play) work, painting, drawing, journaling, psychoeducational reading, dancing, movement and body therapy, group therapy, family therapy, couple therapy, active imagination, and psychodrama. Most analysts would not include body, family, or couple therapy as a part of analysis, although some would. Some Jungian analysts are *very* inclusive about what they consider to be analysis, and others are very exclusive. Jung advocated a broad range of possibility with the understanding that transference inevitably takes place *no matter what,* and that the structure of personality (structure of complexes) is very difficult to affect, that resistance to change is powerful. Different types of people form different types of therapeutic alliance. The analysand should be the guide, not the analyst. The analyst should, however, be well analyzed and able to be reflective and objective about unconscious material.

Methodologically, the two of us are generally non-self-disclosing and moderately expressive, working face-to-face, and very much attuned to a Jungian approach to symbolic interpretation. Dr. Young-Eisendrath considers herself to be in the "developmental school," and Dr. Hall considers himself to be in the "classical school" of Jungian analysis (see Samuels, 1985). The developmental school incorporates clinical–developmental psychology and object relations theory, and it looks rather favorably on a number of Freudian and other psychoanalytic approaches. The developmental school privileges the transferential field and its analysis, somewhat over dream analysis. The classical school uses dream interpretation as the central tool and assumes that dreams will "report" on any disturbances in the transferential field. The classical method includes fewer interpretations of transferential material and more attention simply to dream and symbolic (e.g., symptomatic) material that arises during the course of treatment.

Both of us take an essentially egalitarian attitude toward our analysands and encourage the development of responsibility (for interpretations, for life, work, etc.) within analytic treatment. We both also occasionally (but infrequently) give advice, sometimes assign adjunct reading, and sometimes suggest that our clients attend lectures or workshops (not our own). Dr. Hall uses group psychotherapy as an adjunct to individual treatment with the belief that group work is especially helpful in analyzing the persona and shadow. He coordinates the two in individual treatment.

At the beginning of treatment, Jerry was still palpably attempting to meet his mother-complex standards for being approved. His use of the persona to achieve pseudoacceptance from group members, for instance, permitted him to avoid dealing with the aggressive and enraged shadow (father complex) that actually could have provided motivation and energy. As many men (with puer complexes) believe, Jerry believed that his "real" self (what he sensed as authentic "under the surface") was aggressive and potentially dangerous. The shadow, in other words, seemed to him more authentic than his persona or ego complex, but it had to be hidden away because of its destructive potential, although he would allow it to come out in the very concrete manner of saying "I want to hit you."

Dr. Hall understood the dream of the shop teacher to be a turning point in the early phase of treatment. Catching the fish and hating to kill it (even conversing with it) seemed to reflect a problematic, but ambivalent father complex that is not as aggressive as Jerry feared, but lives far below the surface. Jerry pulled it up from the unconscious (river), and befriended it. The fish speaks when it is treated in this manner. Dr. Hall saw this dream, and some others, as compensations for the aggressive attacks Jerry made on him, and as a development of an attitude of reflection and listening as a result of Dr. Hall's endurance in first being "destroyed" and then "rescued."

Dr. Hall seemed to represent a good father–mother to Jerry, although he was periodically also the abandoning father (in the group) or the critical mother (in refusing to support Jerry's self-pity). As Jerry felt greater access to the good side of the parental complexes, he had the dream of floating into the air within the embrace of the dead father. Jerry interpreted this to mean that it was his *clinging* to the wish for a nurturant father that was his problem. He felt the dream image communicated something like, "If you don't turn loose your yearning (for a good father), you will die." After this dream he felt more hopeful. This hopefulness was expanded by the dream of the refused embrace in the men's restroom; Jerry was again reminded of the inappropriateness of yearning for the embrace of another man; after all, he was himself a father.

It was after this dream that Jerry requested a Mass for his father, although Jerry is not Catholic. He wanted to use the ritual as a means of parting with his father. Again, he moved gradually toward both integration of his own father identity and differentiation from the negative complex. This process is evident in the dream of being with the priest on a high building under construction. The priest, John, awakens a sleeping Jesus figure below. Dr. Hall interpreted this figure as an image of Jerry's self, the central organizing archetype. In another dream soon after, Jerry hears of an imminent execution by "a higher court" that may indicate his self-readiness to dispense with his identification with the youthful persona—the "death" of the dominant puer complex. This kind of death motif can signal a death–rebirth process whereby there is first a dissolution, and then a new integration and differentiation of a subjective state. (Theoretically this is a rearrangement of psychological complexes so that a complex becomes better known, more within self-reflection, less dominant.)

Although Jerry had no other such dreams following these two, he did take the camping trip with his homosexual cousin. Here he had an opportunity to differentiate his complexes and to recognize his anxiety about being homosexual as an intrapsychic situation, not a sexual preference. Testing his own responses and knowing his cousin as a person rather than as a fictive "homosexual" led to differentiation. Things went extremely well, and Jerry began to discriminate the notion of male identity from sexual preference and from the anima (in the form of a mother complex). He felt more comfortable in recognizing that he did not himself have homosexual preferences and in knowing that he could enjoy his cousin and relate to him fully as a man. The visit with the theology professor was yet another occasion of integrating the meaning of male loving. When Dr. O. (private communication from Dr. Hall) told Jerry that he would lend Jerry "ears, heart, and brain," Jerry emphasized the ears. "My own father *never* listened to me," he stressed.

Dr. Hall witnessed the development of greater maturity (e.g., being able to take background as well as foreground roles in the group), of authentic feelings for people unlike himself (e.g., the unkempt neighbor man), and authentic and direct communication in individual therapy. In all of these arenas, Jerry appeared to be less dominated by a need to seek approval, attention, and narcissistic supplies. In other words, the dominance of the negative mother complex (and its accompanying defensive structure of the persona as eternal youth) seemed to recede. At about this time Jerry had the dream of the Devil's Daughter. Dr. Hall's understanding of the dream, at the time of this writing, is that it offers images of a new development in Jerry's personality: the transformation of self into mature man and of anima into sister–lover.

In the dream Jerry attempts to defend himself against the male shadow figure (image of negative father complex) threatening to overwhelm him. When he attempts to take his own power, the anima image invokes the archetypal figure of the Devil. Paradoxically, the anima says she is the daughter of the Devil himself. Her formula for protection (something that Jerry has certainly needed) is presented as a spiky dog. The dog, long associated with defending human territory with the reliable animal instincts of loyalty and shrewdness, is a positive defensive companion for Jerry. Its spikes are perhaps evidence of Jerry's continuing rage, now partly transformed into more assimilable "animal instinct." The dream setting of a theatre suggests the activity of a psychological complex: the repetitive enactments or drama of emotionally charged themes. The anima figure seems confident that she can use this spiky-dog attitude against the most destructive aspects of the Devil, the archetypal negative father. Both the dog and the new anima figure are psychological evidence of Jerry's transformation. As symbols, they provide him with foci for introspection and with motivation for further development. He can (and he has) returned to them again and again to be inspired with his ability to "fight" his negative father complex and to identify with being a father (both positive and negative, but not terrible) himself.

Typical of a classical Jungian analysis, Dr. Hall sees the course of Jerry's treatment affected very much by the emergent symbolization in his dreams, by relationships in the group and with friends and neighbors, *in addition to* the effects of the therapeutic dyad in analysis. The therapeutic dyad is only one "couple" among many that have contributed to Jerry's development of an intrapsychic dialectic.

Dreams are understood to be self-representations of Jerry's psyche with his complexes imaged as the characters and environments with which the dream-self interacts and identifies. As we indicated earlier, Jung insisted that dreams are a natural product of the psyche, neither merely wish nor fantasy, but rather a completion or correction of waking consciousness. By compensating conscious awareness, dreams balance the one-sided experience of subjectivity (i.e., identification with persona or self-representations) that is defended in waking life. Jung asserted that the dream is a text that must be read analogically, not logically (for the most part). Dreams provide us with images of our emotional conflicts and of our ability to develop through them. Unique in their synthetic function, our dreams arouse attention through presenting novel images to convey self-knowledge.

Exploration of Jerry's early history through the analysis of his complexes as they emerged in dreams and other (including therapeutic) relationships revealed the patterns of emotional arousal and cognitive construction that have contributed to Jerry's puer personality. Harsh criticisms and enemas from Mother and a desired but frustrated relationship with Father are the structures that Jerry created and sustained over the years of childhood. As an adult he was unable to part from them. By becoming aware of his limited responsibility for their creation (as a child) and his greater responsibility for their sustenance (as an adult), Jerry is beginning to "stop" believing his complexes as the whole truth, especially the projections onto the valued women and men in his environment.

The ultimate "cure" for the puer complex is work and responsibility-taking. Jerry's major "work" left undone is taking responsibility for his aggressive demands and rage in relating to women. As he has assimilated his identity as an adult male, he has become more available to do this work. Witness his plans to marry and his responsible confrontation with Mother. Obviously as this work is done, and he feels more satisfied with his mature strength, Jerry will (paradoxically) be more able to play, to see his life as providing spontaneous opportunities for pleasure and interest—and not as hopelessly flawed by a flawed past.

The discussion of this case has provided an opportunity to examine Jung's self psychology from a practical viewpoint. In our final chapter, we offer our recommendations for the future. Throughout the book we have alluded to suggestions we would make for the clarification of analytical psychology, especially Jung's self psychology. Finally we have arrived at the point of making them.

☆9☆

The Future?
Recommendations
and Speculations

From the perspective we have gained on Jung's self psychology, we are persuaded that Jung's overall contribution to a theory of subjectivity is uniquely complex and comprehensive. His emphasis on the development of unity over time, through self-reflexivity and differentiation of psychological complexes, is unique in lifespan psychology. Jung clarifies the lifespan development of self beginning with the core being of infancy and later self-recognition, continuing with self-awareness of childhood and early adolescence, developing further through self-reflection of late adolescence and early adulthood, and finally differentiating into a complex self-narrative through the metacognitive recursions of self through later adulthood and aging. More than any other theorist of depth psychology, Jung has identified the processes of symbolic transformation that permit us to recognize and study patterns of individual subjectivity in personal and cultural expressions throughout history and over a lifespan.

The complexity of human subjectivity is daunting. The word "self" seems both too vague and too monolithic to capture this complexity. We believe it is the "right" word, though, for psychological individuality because in common parlance it unifies the subject matter under it. The invariants of subjectivity—agency, coherence, continuity, and emotional arousal—are universally recognized as "self" in whatever cultural form it takes.

In this final chapter, we touch again on several themes we have developed throughout the book. We are particularly interested in clarifying a Jungian epistemology for discourse about self. The first section here is a recommendation for a constructivist theory of self, eliminating certain aspects of Jungian foundationalism or essentialism. Next we make some suggestions and speculations about how other theories of subjectivity—interpersonal and object relations theory, state-dependent theory, dream theory, and Buddhist epistemology—can intersect usefully with Jung's self psychology. We speculate that Jung's self psychology could provide a unifying paradigm for a constructivist psychology of subjectivity and symbolic transformation.

CONSTRUCTIVISM, COMPLEX, AND ARCHETYPE

As we said in Chapter 2, constructivism is an account of things that gives primary status to interpretation, belief, or point of view in understanding an "object" of awareness. Constructivism contends that the world we perceive and experience is not fixed by something "out there" (such as reality, universal forms, or God). Rather, the world is constructed via our embodied interactions with an environment in flux and the aims or purposes of interpretive practices. These interpretive practices emerge in cultural and historical contexts such as society and family. They are not fixed and inflexible, but they are relative to what is held to be "true" or meaningful in any situation. Jung was a radical constructivist in that he believed that the phenomenal world was grounded in *Weltanschauung*—in belief, image, and interpretation.

Jung is often criticized, however, for being a certain kind of realist—a foundationalist or essentialist. His psychology can be seen as a pursuit of universal forms or self-evident givens that arise "out there" and are beyond any context of practice whatsoever. Some of Jung's earliest accounts of self, resting as they do on Kantian metaphysics and Eastern yogic theory, are indeed foundationalist. When Jung talks as though the pattern or structure for self-organization is "given" through a universal or mental category (arising outside of human embodiment), then he is a realist. Moreover, sometimes Jung discusses gender differences and "layers" of the collective unconscious as given, and does indeed apply acultural, ahistorical categories to subjective experiences.

The conflation of levels of analysis in Jungian theory appears to be the problem that interferes most with a constructivist interpretation of self. As we said earlier, Jung tends to blur the distinction between experiential (subjective and intersubjective) and abstract (design or energic) levels of analysis. He fuses the concept of archetypal self (as momentary coherence and organizing principle) with his model of individuation (as the principle of totality, the evolving self as an interrelationship of complexes). This kind of blur becomes a slippery slide from immediate, subjective experience (self/other) to universal pronouncements about the purpose or design of personality that proscribe what is right and natural. This kind of interpretive error creates obstacles to clinical discourse when contextualized experiences (such as gender) are rendered in terms of self-evident givens (such as archetypes of Masculine and Feminine). The error also creates obstacles to larger cultural analyses of symbolic forms when our categories are Eurocentric or otherwise deeply biased.

In taking a constructivist orientation to analytical psychology, we believe that ahistorical, acultural analyses should be eliminated from clinical discourse and that claims for a universal design (individuation) of personality should be understood as hypothetical, reserved for broader theoretical research and study.

In clinical discussions of analytical treatment or psychotherapy with individuals, couples, or families, we recommend a subjective/functional level of analysis. This means that we would confine ourselves to talking about psychological complexes in dialectical relationship, organized to sustain the invariants of self-agency, coherence, continuity, emotional arousal. The organization and experience of a psychological complex depend on emotional–instinctual patterns of human life. The archetypal core or motivating factor is a tendency to form a coherent image in an emotionally aroused state. Certain images belong to that state of arousal, and the reexperiencing of those images or the arousal state may evoke the complex. This affective-imaginal model of psychological complexes is the product of Jung's later (1944–1961) work, and it eliminates his original demarcation between "a collective unconscious" and "a personal unconscious." All psychological complexes are "collective" in the sense that they are motivated by universal (deep structure) instinctual–emotional factors; they are also "personal" in the sense that they comprise the affective particulars, the surface structures, of an individual's experience.

This model of complexes in dialectical relationship is consistent with other contemporary object relations theories such as Sullivan's (1953), Bowlby's (1986), Stern's (1985), Lichtenberg's (1983), and others that describe the evolution of an "inner representational" world through the progressive internalization and differentiation of attachment figures.

Jung does not espouse a "dominance" model of personality development in which one complex (e.g., the ego complex) dominates the entire personality by imposing one symbolic process (e.g., rational-sequential thinking) on all experience. Jung's model of dialectical balance is more "dissociative" in that conscious and unconscious complexes are expected to be in healthy balance when a person feels vitally alive in adulthood.

Jung's self psychology makes the problem of "unity" a central feature of lifespan development. Self-recognition and even self-awareness do not provide unity automatically. Unity is to be understood here as integrity—knowledge of, and responsibility for, the diverse enactments of one's being. Consciousness does not supply a coherent structure for a personality with multiple organizations or multiple voices. The goal of individuation, the development of the self, is unity. That unity can be achieved over a lifetime through a conscious dialectical awareness (insight and reflection on inner conflict) or through accumulated transcendental experiences (transcending ordinary self-images through symbolic expressions or rituals). Unity or the ability to reflect on the totality of one's being is not guaranteed; it is the product of striving in the middle and second half of life. Jung's dissociation model of personality, with individuation as the underlying theoretical design, can speak to such diverse phenomena as hypnotic trance, borderline states, creative inspiration, psychotic episodes, multiple personality, symbolic connections, and neurotic enactments and moods.

Correcting Jung's conflation of self (momentary coherence) and individuation (design of personality), we would specify three levels of analysis for different purposes: design, subjective, and intersubjective. The model of individuation, as the process of self development (especially after the breakdown of the original persona), is a "design strategy" of pattern explanation. Design strategies are used to discuss abstract patterns of organization or structure (see Dennett, 1987). Individuation theory proceeds on the premise that personality has a certain structure or evolving pattern that can be deduced by studying the forms of peoples' symbolic expressions and their transformation over time. Predictions are made that people will behave or emerge developmentally as they were "designed" to do in regard to situational patterns such as attachment, aggression, sexuality, initiation rituals, grief, aging, and the like. Although the theory of individuation can be tested, it is not close to experience or observation. It is hypothetical, and it provides an explanation for development through studying *forms* that are implicit in people's experience, not self-reports or lived life.

Constructivist research in psychology now provides a plausible basis for a theory of individuation that is assumed to be universal or acultural. Contributors such as Piaget, Luria, Vygotsky, Loevinger, Kegan, and Vaillant have provided cross-cultural evidence for a continuum of universal sequencing of different symbolic forms.

At the next level of analysis, the subjective, we encounter the notion of a psychological complex organized around an archetypal core. This would be the "highest" or most abstract level of analysis admissible in clinical discourse. Although we draw on the model of individuation as a premise in terms of the way a person is "supposed" to develop, we would not use design-level (i.e., acultural) explanation. At the subjective level, analysis would follow the function or strategy of a subjective event, paying attention to actual processes and details of personal context. A psychological complex is the primary subjective unit of personality organization from a Jungian perspective. It includes emotional arousal, archetypal images, and personal history.

The affective-imaginal core of a complex is considered "universal" because of the ubiquitous influence of embodiment on perception and emotion. Embodiment theory and research on universal expressions of human emotion provide constructivist frameworks for a theory of archetypes. As we showed in Chapter 2, embodiment theory demonstrates connections between universal epistemological categories and "human-sized" propositional and metaphorical models. Bowlby's working models and Lichtenberg's motivational systems are examples of other constructivist theories of affective-imaginal complexes. The advantage of Jung's theory, in comparison with these others, is its longer life and greater explanatory capacity due to investigations of wide-ranging symbolic expressions over the lifespan. For example, Jung's theory of contrasexual complexes (anima/animus), when presented from a constructivist perspective, provides a revolutionary understanding of the "projection-making factors" that can motivate development of mature subjectivity through the "experiment" of exogamous marriage. Young-Eisendrath (1984) has used this model as the basis for depth psychotherapy with marital couples.

When we limit clinical discourse to the subjective and intersubjective levels of analysis, we automatically correct the misplaced foundationalism in Jung's reasoning. For example, his assumptions of acultural gender differences (that women's consciousness is characterized more by a "connective" quality of Eros and men's more by the "discrimination" of Logos, CW 9, II, p. 14) are a product of the slippery slide from design analysis (the way things are "supposed" to be) to subjective analysis (the experiences of people). If we restrict design analysis to hypothesis-testing in research and theory, then we avoid Jung's mistakes. We recognize that psychological complexes are the products of embodied, lived life. The overall design of selfhood, though, is not part of lived life. Both self and gender are constructions rooted in cultural contexts, organized by a core of affective-imaginal material.

When we talk about the psychological complex of self-images, the ego complex in Jung's terminology, we are faced with the next functional level of analysis, intersubjectivity. With self-recognition comes other-recognition and the gradual organization of subjective and objective experiences. The archetypal self is the motivating core of self-images infused with many emotions, but perhaps especially pride, envy, shame, embarrassment, and guilt—the self-conscious emotions. As we indicated in Chapter 2, psychological complexes organized around the Other are characterized especially by perception or observation rather than direct experience. The psychological Other is gradually discovered to be a psychological individual (a person, like oneself) by recognizing agency, coherence, continuity, and emotional arousal in others around one. The representational world of the Other(s) in the self is organized by emotionally charged complexes (such as Great Mother or Terrible Mother) that are the product of subjective states that will never be completely valid images of actual others.

From a clinical point of view, then, it appears that images of both subjectivity and objectivity reside in the ego complex and other complexes (such as parental complexes and contrasexual complexes). For instance, identifying with a negative Mother complex can evoke configurations of a critical parent and a guilty, powerless child. A person thus alternates between two "voices" and two kinds of affective experiences when overtaken by this complex. Similarly, when a complex is projected onto another person or being in the environment, the other may sound like either the self (perhaps at an earlier stage of development) or an intrapsychic Other. Any therapeutic treatment of the self per se calls forth the full arena of intersubjectivity.

A constructivist interpretation of archetype and complex and the distinction between design and subjective analysis provide a needed corrective for foundationalist tendencies in contemporary uses of analytical psychology. Some therapists and theorists who make use of analytical psychology continue to claim self-evident premises for a sort of Jungian "fairytale" of the psyche. This tale tends to be shaped by Eurocentric ideals and values: each of us has "within" a wise old man/woman, a hero, a divine child, and a trickster. These are frequently called "archetypes of the collective unconscious" and are thought to accompany or overtake the self. The self may be described as though it were a crystalline structure, a mindspace that is almost palpable. A constructivist reading of Jung obviously eliminates this type of acultural, ahistorical discourse from clinical analyses of subjective states.

We hope that these few recommendations for theoretical revision will assist Jungian and other readers in bringing Jung's self psychology into line with contemporary theories of subjectivity and development.

INTERPERSONAL AND OBJECT RELATIONAL THEORIES OF SELF

For our purposes, we consider Harré, Sullivan, Stern, Bowlby, and Kohut to be proponents of an interpersonal self. What we mean is that these theorists centralize the experience of relationship in the process of subjective development. Harré specifically grounds his version of self in the symbiotic relationship. He believes that personal being is primary and that categories of individual psychology are secondary in the development of all people. What Harré adds to Jung's approach is a more careful discrimination of what is universal and what is personal in the psychology of subjectivity. Harré believes that the "moral codes" of personal being and the powers ascribed to persons everywhere are universal in the nature of human life. The degree of psychological individuality, however, is for Harré contingent on the context of society and culture.

Sometimes Jung and Jungians assume a kind of universal psychological individuality and speak about the self as though it were always in the form of strong individualism and personal responsibility. Harré provides a corrective in his examples of some peoples' (e.g., the Copper Eskimo) selves that are more collective, more oriented to group welfare, less competitive, less referenced to individual freedom, etc. Harré adds to Jungian theory a differentiation of the concept of self, grounding it in gender, context, and culture.

Jung adds to Harré the notion of unity or "core being" (see Young-Eisendrath & Hall, 1987, for a full discussion of this). The archetypal self is the potential for individual unity residing in personal being, a unity that can be inferred in the transcendent function of coordinating conscious and unconscious processes. Within the early experiences of the person (in Harré's terms), there must be a potential out of which agency, coherence, continuity, and emotional arousal can eventually develop into self-recognition. Jung calls that potential the "archetypal self."

Stern's model of emergent, core, subjective, and verbal selves is consistent with Jung's theory of archetypal self. Stern's model is very similar to that of Jungian analyst Fordham, as we mentioned earlier. Both Stern and Fordham emphasize the individuality of the self at birth. They also acknowledge the importance of attachment relationships for the progressive and coordinated "de-integration" of the component parts of the individual self. Stern's emergent and core selves depend for development on physical nurturing and emotional mirroring; his subjective self depends on emotional attunements that are interactive and well coordinated between infant and mothering ones.

Stern brings to analytical psychology both an infant research program that is wider ranging than any previous Jungian effort and a restraint about predicating adult functioning on early development. Stern is ecumenical in integrating research from many sources, especially information on affect and perceptual theories. His concept of representations of interactions that have been generalized (RIGs) is wholly consonant with Jung's idea of a psychological complex. Stern's understanding of RIGs in clinical work with adults is an inviting model for Jungians to adopt, especially in reporting case material.

What Jung can add to Stern is a model of psychological individuality developing over a lifetime. Jung was especially good at tracing the process of metacognitive development—from the enactments of complexes to the awareness of them, from awareness to the recognition of compensation and the transcendent function, and then to the acceptance of a central organizing principle for individuality, beyond the ego. This kind of metacognitive orientation is missing in Stern's model and research.

The symbiosis of mother and child is central to Bowlby's model of attachment, separation, and loss, as it is to Harré's notion of personal being. Bowlby's emphasis on the vicissitudes of mother–child interaction can be seen from a Jungian perspective as patterns of mother complexes: secure, anxious, and avoidant. Bowlby's idea of human instinct and of inherent working models resonates well with Jung's theory of archetype and complex. Bowlby's investigations supply necessary empirical evidence for much of Jung's speculation about innate releasing mechanisms and patterning of behavior within archetypal arousal. Jung adds to Bowlby both the emphasis on symbolic process, as noted by Stevens (1982), and the idea that the archetypal configurations of early life develop in relation to the ego complex over a lifetime. Jung emphasizes the symbolizing function of human instinctual responses. Bowlby emphasizes action patterns organized around core affects.

Bowlby appears to be a determinist in the way he sees the effects of early patterns (secure, avoidant, resistant) of attachment on later personality patterns of adulthood. Jung emphasizes rather the restructuring of personality at different phases of the lifespan. As we indicated in Chapter 2, Jung believed that self-division through psychological conflict opened the door to new developmental possibilities. From Jung's point of view, a happy and secure childhood does not necessarily lead to healthy development in adulthood. Because neurotic conflict is seen by

Jung to be a necessary step in the development of later self-reflexivity, he does not privilege happiness or security in childhood.

Jung's vision of the self in evolution (rather than as a static pattern) is, of course, similar to Sullivan's idea that the self-system can be revised with each new developmental period. Sullivan's self-system per se is comparable more to the Jungian idea of persona than it is to the self or ego complex. Sullivan's self-system is a structure of security operations, used to protect oneself from the disintegrating tension of anxiety. Jung's persona is a defensive presentation, a "mask" that both reveals and hides the actor. Jung believes the persona serves a useful function both in the development of the personality and in momentary interactions. This function is to preserve coherence when a person does not experience coherence. Sullivan, on the other hand, has an entirely negative view of the self-system, in the sense that it acts as a barrier to intimacy and tends to perpetuate selective inattention and resistance to change.

Sullivan's strong interpersonal emphasis on modes of prototaxic, parataxic, and syntaxic organization matches well with Jung's archetypal, complex, and personal modes or realities (see Young-Eisendrath, 1985, for a complete discussion). Both theorists emphasize that none of these modes can be reduced to another, that they are wholly distinct and different methods of constructing worlds and communicating. Clinically, we must recognize them as different languages or semiotic systems.

Sullivan provides a new lens for a Jungian theory of psychological complexes. Sullivan moves our understanding of psychological complexes fully into the interpersonal field, the relational space of projection and projective identification. This lens adds much to the analysis of transference and countertransference when psychological complexes are "discharged" into the therapeutic relationship. They can be seen as organizing the relational dynamics between analysand and analyst, rather than simply arising in one or another. From Sullivan's viewpoint, both analysand and analyst will organize themselves defensively to avoid anxiety. The location and measure of anxiety are important indicators of the attitude or mode (prototaxic, parataxic, syntaxic) that is employed to grasp what is taking place.

Jung's self psychology also adds much to a Sullivanian approach to subjectivity. Jung's emphasis on unity and its development, on forms of symbolic transformation, and on the universal organization of the self provide "integrating" tendencies that are different from basic needs. Sullivan's self-system functions only as a defensive maneuver to avoid anxiety in interpersonal negotiations. Sullivan does not advance a theory of self that matches his relational concept of "intimacy" as the goal of mature development. Jung's theory of affective-imaginal life is largely compatible with a Sullivanian approach and supplements Sullivan's rather narrow view of self. Jung's model of contrasexuality in self development provides the missing link in Sullivan's theory of intimacy.

Kohut's understanding of self and self-object is similar to Jung's, but it is more relational than intrapsychic. Kohut, like Bowlby, tends to stress the parents' functions as self-objects in a way that might lead us to believe that early needs predominate over later ones developmentally.

Kohut acknowledges that all parents fail to meet self-object needs in their children and that this failure should be "optimal" for development, or narcissistic wounds will appear in later deficits in the ability to sustain self-love. Developmental failures actually provide the means for modulating the inflation of self and self-objects. The optimal balance of narcissistic resources in self and parental other, and failures of these resources, paves the way to healthy and stable functioning.

This Kohutian framework for understanding and treating psychological inflation provides a useful interpersonal antidote to Jung's entirely intrapsychic analysis of identification of ego complex with self, or self with ego. Moreover, Kohut's attention to the need for therapeutic empathy and for mature dependence on self-objects is a useful addition to Jung's more alchemical and symbolic understanding of transference. Many Jungian theorists and clinicians have drawn substantially on Kohut's analyses of self in explaining the influence of parental complexes on adult self-esteem. Fewer have incorporated the interpersonal framework of Kohut's approach in the therapeutic setting.

A Jungian orientation to Kohut's self psychology completes the picture of subjective development by filling out a model for transformation in adult life. Jung's model of contrasexual complexes, connecting self and world (see Chapter 5), is a version of self and the self-object relationship that evolves from enactments (in adolescence and early adulthood) to symbolizations in middle and later adulthood. Jung's account emphasizes the projection-making factor of intrapsychic functioning, but it recognizes that psychological movement into culture and world is the occasion for differentiation when projections are resisted by others and then understood.

Much more could be said about the correspondence and complementarity between Jungian theory and object relations theory. We leave the topic here, but we assume our readers have made other connections from the detailed accounts we presented in Chapter 7. Overall, Jung's self psychology appears to be an overarching paradigm that can assimilate other models of the inner representational world. Analytical psychology benefits from the more interpersonal emphases of many of these models, and the object relational framework is enhanced through being connected to Jung's grander program of individuation.

CONTEMPORARY DREAM SCIENCE
AND JUNGIAN THEORY

In Allan Hobson's *The Dreaming Brain* (1988), he reviews empirical dream research from the early work of the Spanish histologist Ramon y Cajal and his discovery of discrete brain neurons to the recent discoveries of Mircea Steriade of Quebec, who has been instrumental in helping us understand the nature of brain states that accompany dreaming. Hobson claims that his own "activation-synthesis" model of dreaming is similar to Jung's dream theory, but Hobson is wrong. Although Hobson says his theory "echoes Jung's notion of dreams as transparently meaningful and does away with any distinction between manifest and latent content" (p. 12), he actually offers a model that reduces mind to brain, and dreaming to brain mechanisms and vegetative life. The obvious conclusion from Hobson's model is that dreaming is another form of "information processing." Jung, as has been amply shown, never reasons reductively about instinct, image, or symbol.

Hobson's book provides a creditable review of modern dream science, however, and in this way is significant in supporting Jung's theory of a transcendent function that balances or compensates waking and sleeping life. Sleep provides us with the opportunity to dream, and dreaming provides us with the possibility of resolving emotional conflicts without endangering ourselves or others. Jung, of course, insisted that the dream was a natural product of the psyche, rather than a neurotic production of latent wishes. From his own analysis and his clinical work, he came to the notion of the transcendent function. Dreaming, as experienced in sleep, presents a version of self-knowledge that transcends our ordinary subjectivity, our individual self. The dream, as remembered, is a text in which appear image and symbol, narrating ourselves. These depict—as a straightforward communication in a language different from the sequential language of waking life—our emotional conflicts and our ability to develop through them.

Probably best known among dream scientists are Nathaniel Kleitman and Eugene Aserinsky who, in 1953, reported in *Science* magazine their discovery of patterns of eye movement and cortical arousal during sleep. It is now common knowledge that what is usually called a "dream" occurs 90–95% of the time in a brain state characterized by high cortical arousal and rapid movement of the eyes. Rapid eye movement (REM) sleep has almost become synonymous with dreaming, although there are some dreams in non-rapid-eye-movement (non-REM) sleep as well. The kind of dreaming that Jung and Freud studied, and the kind that people typically report on waking and in psychotherapy, is the REM type. All of us are in REM sleep about 25% of our sleeping time—that is about 6 years of a 70-year lifespan—during which we are probably having dreams that fit the following ubiquitous pattern:

1. Narrative construction, plot, story form.
2. Emotional arousal (sometimes intense emotion).
3. Disruptions of ordinary subjectivity—of the experiences of embodiment, agency, coherence, and continuity as we usually expect them.
4. Uncritical acceptance of these disruptions with little or no self-reflection.
5. Vivid, fully formed, and perceived images—primarily visual, but also auditory, tactile, kinesthetic (rarely gustatory or olfactory, even more rarely physically painful).
6. Difficulty remembering the dream upon waking, especially after moving about and thinking other thoughts.

Beginning in the 1960s, laboratory and home documentation of human sleep cycles (for example, the work of physiologist Wilse Webb) has shown that REM sleep comes in three or four bouts for all of us, lasting from a few minutes to about an hour each. Neurophysiologist Mircea Steriade of Quebec has been instrumental in helping us understand the brain states associated with dreaming. REM sleep is the result of increased activation of REM-on neurons in the brain stem (reticular activating system) that can be turned on only as a result of deepest sleep (when certain other REM-off neurons are deactivated). Although Freud believed that the dream was the guardian of sleep—protecting us from being jarred awake by anxiety-provoking wishes—it now appears that sleep (especially the state of deepest sleep) is the guardian of the dream, permitting the brain state in which dreaming can occur.

From our above description of the REM dream, we can easily see that dreaming disrupts three of the four invariants of subjectivity. Only emotional arousal—the patterning of affective experiencing and expressing—links sleeping, dreaming, and waking life. When personal subjectivity is inhibited by sleep but emotions are aroused, dreams will provide the images and symbols that excite our curiosity and confront us with self-knowledge. The intense cortical involvement and the amount of time committed to dreaming imply that dreaming is important to survival.

It appears that dreaming gives image and expression to the psychological complexes that grip us in daily life, especially those that disturb our balance or unity. That dreams are hard to remember (even in dream laboratories) may indicate that they are meant to provide their correctives primarily while we are sleeping. Hence, they provide a recursive loop of self-knowledge that can affect our actions without our knowing it. Dream science supports Jung's idea of a transcendent function: Each of us every night is intensely aroused by self-knowledge that is an antidote to the egocentrism of waking life. Jung's psychology of self and transcendent function could provide a theory for contemporary dream science that is neither reductionistic nor materialistic, that doesn't reduce dreaming to brain functions.

STATE-DEPENDENT LEARNING
AND PSYCHOLOGICAL COMPLEXES

In various ways, both Ernest Rossi (1986) and Morton Reiser (1984) call on the notion of "state-dependent" learning or memory in an effort to unite contemporary neurobiological theories and the emotional reenactments of psychotherapy. Reiser wants to clarify how a psychological complex can be organized over time and reexperienced as a trance-like state in psychoanalysis. He turns especially to the physiology of stress and memory. Rossi is more direct, however, in discussing the particular theory of state-dependent learning. Rossi wants to substantiate a theory for hypnotic trance. Quoting from his own work with Milton Erickson, Rossi says,

> Inasmuch as experience arises from the binding or coupling of a particular state or level of arousal with a particular symbolic interpretation of that arousal, experience is state-bound; thus, it can be evoked either by inducing the particular level of arousal, or by presenting some symbol of its interpretation, such as an image, melody, or taste. (p. 40)

Rossi goes on to suggest even that the apparent continuity that exists in personal subjectivity is "in fact a precarious illusion" because it is made possible only by the associative connections that relate bits of conversation and task orientation.

The theory of state-dependent learning—that we have categorized or collected our experiences into emotion-laden meaning systems—is strongly supportive of Jung's theory of psychological complexes. In the hypnosis literature and in studies of altered states of consciousness, as well as ordinary memory, the theme of state dependence is broadly illustrated with both laboratory and case studies. Rossi (1986) attempts to link state dependence and the whole system of mind–body connection through the limbic model of the mind and the process of memory storage and retrieval. Rossi wants to establish a nondualistic theory of mind–

action to support clinical hypnosis as a treatment method and a form of investigation. Reiser (1984) attempts something similar in using psychoanalytic metapsychology and clinical theory to illustrate the neurobiological models of hormonal/affective/cognitive systems.

Jung made us aware of the fundamental dissociative nature of personality by advancing his model of psychological complexes, and in this way he presaged the study of state-dependent learning. The interface between his theory of psychological complexes and research on state-dependent learning is fruitful both empirically and clinically. Empirically, we may discover something about the cognitive nature of affective-imaginal life, the link between mood and organized experience, between feelings and memories. Clinically, we gain much from the analogy of hypnotic trance or state-dependent events and the experience of being in a psychological complex.

PHILOSOPHY OF BUDDHISM
AND JUNG'S SELF THEORY

Buddhism (as established originally through the teachings of Gautama Buddha, approximately 2,500 years ago) is a pragmatic set of instructions for daily life that is both an epistemology and an ontology, although it is not a metaphysical ontology.

Buddhism provides a method of systematic analysis of conventional and metaphysical knowledge; it is similar in many ways to contemporary constructivism and forms of psycholinguistic analysis. Buddhist epistemological analysis is used specifically to "undo" metaphysics and not to create meta-thinking. Buddhism is also a practice or discipline of daily life that is designed to free one from "obsessions" and to preserve a middle path between conflicting opposites. In this way it is similar to contemporary psychotherapy.

Drawing especially on the second-century Indian philosopher Nagarjuna, whose work is presented in translation and with commentary by Kalupahana (1986), we want to present a few of the major tenets of Buddhism because they further clarify a constructivist approach to Jung's self psychology. As Kalupahana says,

> The survival of a pragmatic philosophy in the face of an extremely absolutistic tradition such as the one embodied in the *Bhagavadgita* was not easy. . . . The Buddhist philosophers, confronted by the onslaught of Indian thinkers asserting the reality of self. . . . spent most of their time analysing what they called *dhamma* in order to show that there was no permanent and eternal self. (p. 20)

The concept of *dhamma* means roughly "anything that is given in experience" or phenomenal reality.

The following is a brief example of a Buddhist analysis of the function of language in relation to *dhamma*. In Buddhist principles, all phenomenal experience rests on consciousness. Form and matter, sensation, perception, and psychological disposition are the composite elements of consciousness. According to Buddhist epistemological constraints, language must not "cling to dialectical usage nor go beyond the limits of linguistic convention" (p. 19). Language is assumed to be neither ultimately real (in terms of depicting some "reality" such as time or space) nor ultimately useless in expressing reality. Language derives its meaning through the results it produces. Linguistic expressions that imply permanence or impermanence of the phenomenal world do not communicate anything that is given in experience *(dhamma)*, and so they are false.

A good deal of Buddhist analysis of conventional thinking and metaphysics proceeds in the above manner to decide whether a statement is true or false when it is constrained by *dhamma*. All conventions of thinking and all constructions of reality depend on specific conditions. None of them is absolute and ultimate; they are all subject to change.

Analysis leads to "freedom" from obsessional thinking in that a person learns not to believe conventional truths but rather to understand their conditionality and their useful significance without elevating them to an ultimate. Obsession is the tendency to argue for or against such truths. According to Buddhist accounts of it, resisting this tendency is more difficult than abandoning the pleasures of the sensory world.

Dogmatism in any form, whether it is nihilism or absolutism, is the problem that Buddhist analysis confronts. Dogmatism leads to conflicts among human beings, according to the Buddha, and to wars, destruction of the environment, and the like.

Buddhism is a philosophy of the "middle way," one that does not adhere to any dogma. One discovers the perspective of the middle way through actions that it engenders. This perspective leads to the core concept of Buddhist ontology: compassion is "right action." Self-restraint and benefiting others are the actions that naturally emerge in a person who is successfully practicing the philosophy of Buddhism.

Like constructivism, Buddhism attends mainly to effects of belief and interpretation on constructions of reality. In regard to self psychology, the belief in a permanent or eternal self produces such ideas as "inner control" and a reified or substantial self. This kind of belief is shown to be context-dependent, and hence only a theory that arises under specific conditions that engender it.

In the formal teachings of this philosophy, there is no attempt to resolve the issue of whether or not a self exists, but rather, there is simply an examination of the context in which the belief arises. In a sense, Buddhist analysis leads away from drawing sharp metaphysical distinctions and toward understanding circumstantial meanings.

As we alluded in Chapter 7, Buddhist epistemology adds something to Jung's notion of synchronicity by stressing the fact that phenomenal experience is always dependent on context and circumstances for its meaning and reality. Experience does not exist apart from the consciousness of its substantiality. In this way, the phenomenal experience of an emotion-laden image depends on the context in which it arises, just as other images depend on the intersubjective world in which they arise. From a Buddhist point of view, images that arise in core emotional states are "real" as much as the phenomenal world is real. Buddhists do not privilege the material world as the generator of phenomena. They take the position that all phenomena are dependent on a context for their substantiation and leave it at that.

Buddhist analysis supports Jungian constructivism in its insistence on opposing the reification of the self. By restoring contextual analysis to understanding subjectivity, the Buddhist position goes around the metaphysical arguments about an essential self. Instead of arguing for or against a foundational self, one always returns to the context (family, culture, transferential field of therapy) in which the self is constructed in order to understand how that particular version of self arose.

Similarly, Buddhism resists *all* ultimate explanations with a firm refusal to argue their inherent meanings (either for or against). Knowledge arises out of contexts, and its use is dependent on them. Buddhist epistemology sounds very much like contemporary constructivism. As Kalupahana (1986) puts it,

> A living human being needs to act. Action involves understanding. Conduct is preceded by knowledge. One needs knowledge of oneself and the external world. "Omniscience" or knowledge of everything was not available to the Buddha. Hence, neither the absolute origin of things nor the absolute end of things was discussed in Buddhism . . . Any theory that attempts to explain such origins and ends, whether it pertains to an eternal self or soul . . . or a substance . . . was unacceptable to the Buddha. (p. 219)

In our discussion of the conflation of subjectivity and design levels of analysis, we touched on the problem of Jungian "omniscience," the tendency to name universals that are beyond experience. We believe that this tendency is a mistake arising out of Jung's refusal to constrain his theory of subjectivity according to a systematic program based on his premise of affective-imaginal construction of meaning.

We have added a Buddhist epistemology here in order to show how a traditional and strong epistemology of constructivism would handle the implications of first premises. We believe that Jung's self psychology benefits on all levels, from subjectivity to synchronicity, from a thorough-going contextual definition of the archetypal self as an organizing tendency arising in a situational context.

FINAL CRITIQUE AND A FEW RECOMMENDATIONS

Because Jung was intrigued by the possibility of designing a vast integrative model—a psychological account of the entire phenomenal world—he was tempted to speculate about the divine, the "designer" of the design strategy. His study of Job is one such speculation. Through this study, he discovered something about the evolution of consciousness in the human personality and the mutual interdependence of unconsciousness and consciousness. His tendency, however, to describe or name what is beyond experience is at odds with a constructivist program. What is beyond experience can be inferred through studying form and pattern, but it cannot be known.

Related to this problem is some tendency in Jung to "know" what is right and natural, to confuse archetype with stereotype. His attempt to erect ideal models for personality functioning that encompass such relative functions as gender, achievement in the world, nurturance, or spontaneity is neither scientifically responsible nor psychologically useful. Jung and Jungians sometimes unintentionally use stereotypes to talk about feelings, spontaneity, idealism, or nurturance (usually based on European or American culture) and call these "archetypes," asserting that they are universally true for all people.

This can result in a kind of theorizing in which women and men are cast into rigidly defined roles for behavior and lifespan development. Even worse, it can lead to occasions in which stereotyped images of people are used to symbolize aspects of the psyche (e.g., a nude woman as the anima). It is not merely that these figures are discussed as images of psychological complexes but, rather, that they are proffered to represent some "essential" state of mind.

Some Jungian characterizations of the anima and the shadow are indeed European stereotypes. Examples of these stereotypes are well-documented in Sander Gilman's (1985) study of stereotypes of sexuality, race, and madness.

The desire to maintain the coherence of self or group leads to stereotyping others, says Gilman. Stereotyping of the outsider (the mad person, the woman, the African–American) is "double-edged." It takes shape both in positive idealized images and in negative devalued ones.

> The "pathological" may appear as the pure, the unsullied; the sexually different as the apotheosis of beauty, the asexual or the androgynous; the racially different as highly attractive. . . . Categories of difference are protean, but they appear as absolutes. They categorize the sense of the self, but establish an order—the illusion of order in the world. (Gilman, 1985, p. 25)

When categories of difference—gender, racial, and ethnic—appear as absolutes, then we have reason to be concerned about how these differences are being used to defend a sense of order.

In Jungian psychology, some gender (masculine/feminine) and racial stereotypes have been used to characterize a manner (e.g., logical) or a psychological complex (e.g., the shadow). Jung also argued that autonomous complexes, our sub-personalities, should be described as living beings in order to be true to our experiences. To represent the shadow as a black man or the anima as a blond, shapely woman obviously encourages stereotypes of race and gender that are wrong and harmful.

If an individual dreams about a black man, the image must be contextualized in the experiences and feelings of the dreamer, not interpreted automatically as the shadow complex. If a man has fantasies about a blond, shapely woman, the fantasies are to be seen in the light of his male anima, not as a portrayal of what it's like to be such a woman. All of these distinctions are clarified by a constructivist approach that does not permit the reifying of psychological complexes and archetypes.

Our vision for a constructivist version of Jung's self psychology is of an overarching theoretical framework for aspects of object relations theory, state-dependent learning, various dissociation models of personality, and certain models for metacognitive processes, such as stage theories. Using the concepts of compensation and transcendent function, as well as archetype and complex, theorists and practitioners would be able to integrate and systematize a number of ideas about psychological processes that are not now a part of a larger theory.

With the improved recording of clinical cases by Jungian and other therapists, and the clarification of the interpersonal field (and our ability to report on it), we should be able to study issues of subjectivity and intersubjectivity in an increasingly precise and comprehensive way.

It is our hope that analytical psychology can be examined more objectively and studied more empirically in the coming decades. As we have tried to show, the theory provides a working model that is both conceptually broad and uniquely well articulated through cross-cultural references. Jung's theory of self is a dialectical model of the development of subjectivity through the differentiation and integration of psychological complexes. It is an attempt to explain the underlying function that permits all embodied persons to recognize themselves as coherent, continuous, and emotionally roused agents, who sustain their purposes through self-reflection.

The model of Jung's self psychology that we advocate here is a revision in line with his own last works. We do not consider our constructivist perspective to be a major shift away from the program of Jung's final contributions to a theory of subjectivity. Rather, we consider this approach to be an enhancement of the orientation Jung was using at the time of his death. Foundationalism, stereotyping, and Eurocentric bias have been barriers to incorporating analytical psychology into contemporary depth psychology and object relations theories. Our approach clarifies these difficulties and resolves them in the overall context of pattern explanation and constructivist epistemology.

Jung was a prolific writer and a visionary thinker. His notion of psychological development indeed established a new and different *Weltanschauung* from the rational empiricism of his day. If we can make use of his understanding of a psychological dialectic and incorporate his model of affective-imaginal life, we may discover a more precise model for subjectivity developing over the lifespan. This would be a model that would represent conflict as consciousness and symptom as symbol and would recognize the self as the knowledge that comes from suffering. In a letter written in 1945, Jung phrased the essence of his model thus:

> You yourself are a conflict that rages in itself and against itself, in order to melt its incompatible substances . . . in the fire of suffering, and thus create that fixed and unalterable form which is the goal of life. Everyone goes through this mill, consciously or unconsciously, voluntarily or forcibly. (Jung, 1973b, p. 375)

References

Aserinsky, E., & Kleitman, N. (1953). Regularly occurring periods of eye motility and concurrent phenomena during sleep. *Science, 118,* 273–274.

Bateson, G. (1972). *Steps to an ecology of mind.* New York: Ballantine.

Belenky, M. F., Clinchy, B. M., Goldberger, N. R., & Tarule, J. M. (1986). *Women's ways of knowing: The development of self, voice, and mind.* New York: Basic Books.

Bellah, R. N., Madsen, R., Sullivan, W. M., Swidler, A., & Tipton, S. M. (1985). *Habits of the heart: Individualism and commitment in American life.* New York: Harper & Row.

Beth, E. W., & Piaget, J. (1966). *Epistemologic mathematique et psychologie.* Paris: Presses Universitaires de France.

Blofeld, J. (1977). *Bodhisattva of compassion: The mystical tradition of Kuan Yin.* Boston: Shambhala.

Bower, G. (1981). Mood and memory. *American Psychologist, 36,* 129–148.

Bowlby, J. (1969). *Attachment and loss* (Vol. 1). London: Hogarth Press.

Bowlby, J. (1986). *Developmental psychiatry comes of age: The 1986 Adolf Meyer lecture.* London: Tavistock Clinic.

Broughton, J. (1987). Piaget's concept of the self. In P. Young-Eisendrath & J. Hall (Eds.), *The book of the self* (pp. 277–295). New York: New York University Press.

Bruner, J. (1986). *Actual minds, possible worlds.* Cambridge, MA: Harvard University Press.

Campbell, J. (1968). *The hero with a thousand faces.* Princeton, NJ: Princeton University Press.

Chomsky, N. (1957). *Syntactic structures.* The Hague: Morton.

Chomsky, N. (1975). *Reflections on language.* New York: Pantheon.

Colby, A., & Kohlberg, L. (1987). *The measurement of moral judgment: A manual and its results.* Cambridge, England: Cambridge University Press.

Costa, P. T., McCrae, R. R., & Arenberg, D. (1983). Recent longitudinal research on personality and aging. In K. W. Schaie (Ed.), *Longitudinal studies of adult psychological development* (pp. 222–265). New York: Guilford Press.

Coward, H. (1985). *Jung and Eastern thought.* Albany, NY: SUNY Press.

171

Csikszentmihalyi, M., & Larson, R. (1984). *Being adolescent: Conflict and growth in the teenage years.* New York: Basic Books.

DeCharms, R. (1968). *Personal causation: The internal affective determinants of behavior.* New York: Academic Press.

Dennett, D. (1987). *The intentional stance.* Cambridge, MA: MIT Press.

Dyson, F. (1988). *Infinite in all directions.* New York: Harper & Row.

Eagle, M. (1984). *Recent developments in psychoanalysis: A critical evaluation.* New York: McGraw-Hill.

Edelson, M. (1984). *Hypothesis and evidence in psychoanalysis.* Chicago: University of Chicago Press.

Ellenberger, H. F. (1970). *The discovery of the unconscious.* New York: Basic Books.

Fairbairn, W. R. (1952). *Psychoanalytic studies of the personality.* Boston: Routledge & Kegan Paul.

Fairbairn, W. R. (1954). *An object relations theory of the personality.* New York: Basic Books.

Fordham, M. (1969). *Children as individuals.* London: Hodder & Stoughton.

Fordham, M. (1985). *Exploration into the self.* London: Academic Press.

Freud, S. (1953a). The interpretation of dreams. In J. Strachey (Ed. and Trans.), *The standard edition of the complete psychological works of Sigmund Freud* (Vols. 4 & 5). London: Hogarth Press. (Original work published in 1905)

Freud, S. (1953b). Three essays on the theory of sexuality. In J. Strachey (Ed. and Trans.), *The standard edition of the complete psychological works of Sigmund Freud* (Vol. 7). London: Hogarth Press. (Original work published in 1905)

Freud, S. (1959). Inhibitions, symptoms and anxiety. In J. Strachey (Ed. and Trans.), *The standard edition of the complete psychological works of Sigmund Freud* (Vol. 21). London: Hogarth Press. (Original work published in 1926)

Freud, S. (1961). The ego and the id. In J. Strachey (Ed. and Trans.), *The standard edition of the complete psychological works of Sigmund Freud* (Vol. 19). London: Hogarth Press. (Original work published in 1923)

Gedo, J. (1979). *Beyond interpretation: Toward a revised theory of psychoanalysis.* New York: International University Press.

Gilligan, C. (1982). *In a different voice: Psychological theory and women's development.* Cambridge, MA: Harvard University Press.

Gilman, S. (1985). *Difference and pathology: Stereotypes of sexuality, race, and madness.* Ithaca, NY: Cornell University Press.

Golan, N. (1986). *The perilous bridge: Helping clients through mid-life transitions.* New York: The Free Press.

Goodheart, W. (1980). Theory of analytic interaction. *The San Francisco Jung Institute Library Journal* (Vol. 1).

Gould, S. J. (1987). *Time's arrow, time's cycle.* Cambridge, MA: Harvard University Press.

Greenberg, J. R., & Mitchell, S. A. (1983). *Object relations in psychoanalytic theory.* Cambridge, MA: Harvard University Press.

Grünbaum, A. (1984). *The foundation of psychoanalysis: A philosophical critique.* Berkeley, CA: University of California Press.

Guidano, V. F. (1987). *The complexity of the self.* New York: Guilford Press.

Guidano, V. F., & Liotti (1983). *Cognitive processes and emotional disorders: A structural approach to psychotherapy.* New York: Guilford Press.

Hall, J. (1977). *Clinical uses of dreams: Jungian interpretations and enactments.* New York: Grune & Stratton.

Hall, J. A. (1989). *Hypnosis: A Jungian perspective.* New York: Guilford Press.

Harré, R. (1984). *Personal being.* Cambridge, MA: Harvard University Press.

Harré, R. (1989). The "self" or a theoretical concept. In M. Krausz (Ed.), *Relativism: Interpretation and confrontation.* Notre Dame, IN: University of Notre Dame Press. 387–417.

Hartmann, H. (1958). *Ego psychology and the problem of adaptation.* New York: International Universities Press. (Original work published 1939)

Hobson, A. (1988). *The dreaming brain.* New York: Basic Books.

Holt, R. R. (1984). *The current status of psychoanalytic theory.* Address presented at the meeting of the American Psychological Association, Toronto.

Izard, C. (1977). *Human emotions.* New York: Plenum Press.

Jacobson, E. (1964). *The self and the object world.* New York: International Universities Press.

Johnson (1987). *The body in the mind: The bodily basis of meaning, imagination, and reason.* Chicago: University of Chicago Press.

Jung, C. G. (1953, 1966). *The collected works of C. G. Jung: Two essays on analytical psychology* (Vol. 7) (R. F. C. Hull, Trans.). Princeton, NJ: Princeton University Press.

Jung, C. G. (1953–1979). *The collected works* (Bollingen Series XX, 20 Vols., R. F. C. Hull, Trans.; H. Read, M. Fordham, G. Adler, & W. McGuire, Eds.). Princeton, NJ: Princeton University Press.

Jung, C. G. (1956). *The collected works of C. G. Jung: Symbols of transformation* (Vol. 5) (R. F. C. Hull, Trans.). Princeton, NJ: Princeton University Press.

Jung, C. G. (1959). *The collected works of C. G. Jung: Aion* (2nd ed., Vol. 9, Part II) (R. F. C. Hull, Trans.). Princeton, NJ: Princeton University Press.

Jung, C. G. (1961). *Memories, dreams, reflections* (rev. ed.). New York: Vintage Books.

Jung, C. G. (1966). *The collected works of C. G. Jung: The practice of psychotherapy* (Vol. 16) (R. F. C. Hull, Trans.). Princeton, NJ: Princeton University Press.

Jung, C. G. (1967). *The collected works of C. G. Jung: Alchemical studies* (Vol. 13) (R. F. C. Hull, Trans.). Princeton, NJ: Princeton University Press.

Jung, C. G. (1969a). *The collected works of C. G. Jung: The archetypes and the collective unconscious* (2nd ed., Vol. 9, Part I) (R. F. C. Hull, Trans.). Princeton, NJ: Princeton University Press.

Jung, C. G. (1969b). *The collected works of C. G. Jung: The structure and dynamics of the psyche* (2nd ed., Vol. 8) (R. F. C. Hull, Trans.). Princeton, NJ: Princeton University Press.

Jung, C. G. (1969c). *The collected works of C. G. Jung: Psychology and religion: East and West* (Vol. 11) (R. F. C. Hull, Trans.). Princeton, NJ: Princeton University Press.

Jung, C. G. (1970). *The collected works of C. G. Jung: Civilization in transition* (Vol. 10) (R. F. C. Hull, Trans.). Princeton, NJ: Princeton University Press.

Jung, C. G. (1971). *The collected works of C. G. Jung: Psychological types* (Vol. 6) (H. G.

Boynes, Trans.; Revised by R. F. C. Hull). Princeton, NJ: Princeton University Press.

Jung, C. G. (1973a). *The collected works of C. G. Jung: Experimental researches* (Vol. 2) (L. Stein, Trans.). Princeton, NJ: Princeton University Press.

Jung, C. G. (1973b). *Letters: 1906–1950*. Princeton, NJ: Princeton University Press.

Jung, C. G. (1975). *Letters: 1951–1961*. Princeton, NJ: Princeton University Press.

Jung, C. G. (1976). *The collected works of C. G. Jung: The symbolic life* (Vol. 18) (R. F. C. Hull, Trans.). Princeton, NJ: Princeton University Press.

Kalupahana, D. (1986). *Nāgārjuna: The philosophy of the middle way*. Albany, NY: SUNY Press.

Kegan, R. (1982). *The evolving self*. Cambridge, MA: Harvard University Press.

Keller, E. F. (1985). *Reflections on gender and science*. New Haven, CT: Yale University Press.

Kernberg, O. F. (1976). *Object-relations theory and clinical psychoanalysis*. Northvale, NJ: Jason Aronson.

Kohlberg, L. (1981). *The philosophy of moral development*. New York: Harper & Row.

Kohut, H. (1971). *The analysis of the self*. New York: International Universities Press.

Kohut, H. (1977). *The restoration of the self*. New York: International Universities Press.

Kohut, H. (1984). *How does analysis cure?* Chicago: University of Chicago Press.

Lakoff, G. (1987). *Women, fire, and dangerous things: What categories reveal about the mind*. Chicago: University of Chicago Press.

Lakoff, G., & Johnson, M. (1980). *Methaphors we live by*. Chicago: University of Chicago Press.

Levinson, D. J., Darrow, C. N., Klein, E. B., Levinson, M. H., & McKee, B. (1978). *The seasons of a man's life*. New York: Knopf.

Lewis, H. B. (1988). Freudian theory and new information in modern psychology. *Psychoanalytic Psychology, 5*(1), 7–22.

Lewis, M., Sullivan, M. W., Stanger, C., & Weiss, M. (1989). Self-development and self-conscious emotions. *Child Development, 60*, 146–156.

Lichtenberg, J. (1983). *Psychoanalysis and infant research*. Hillsdale, NJ: Analytic Press.

Lichtenberg, J. (1989). *Psychoanalysis and motivation*. Hillsdale, NJ: Analytic Press.

Loevinger, J. (1976). *Ego development*. San Francisco: Jossey-Bass.

Loevinger, J., & Wessler, R. (1970). *Measuring ego development I: Construction and use of a sentence completion test*. San Francisco: Jossey-Bass.

Luria, A. A. (1979). *The making of mind: A personal account of soviet psychology* (M. Cole & S. Cole, Eds.). Cambridge, MA: Harvard University Press.

MacMurray, J. (1961). *Persons in relation*. Atlantic Highlands, NJ: Humanities Press.

Mahler, M., Pine, F., & Bergman, A. (1975). *The psychological birth of the infant: Symbiosis and individuation*. New York: Basic Books.

Maturana, H., & Varela, F. (1980). *Autopoiesis and cognition: The realization of the living*. Boston: D. Reidel.

Money, J. (1976). Differentiation of gender identity. *JSAS Catalog of Selected Documents in Psychology, 6(4)*.

Nagel, T. (1986). *The view from nowhere*. New York: Oxford University Press.

Neumann, E. (1954). *The origins and history of consciousness*. Princeton, NJ: Princeton University Press.

Overton, W. (1989). Piaget: The logic of creativity and the creativity of logic. *Contemporary Psychology, 34*(7), 629–631.

Overton, W. (1990). The structure of developmental theory. In P. van Geert & L. P. Moss (Eds.), *Annals of theoretical psychology*. New York: Plenum.

Overton, W. F., Ward, S. L., Noveck, I., Black, J., & O'Brien, D. P. (1987). Form and content in the development of deductive reasoning. *Developmental Psychology, 23*, 22–30.

Perry, W. (1970). *Forms of intellectual and ethical development in the college years*. New York: Holt, Rinehart & Winston.

Perry, H. S., (1981). *The psychiatrist of America*. Cambridge, MA: Harvard University Press.

Piaget, J. (1926). *The language and thought of the child* (M. Warden, Trans.). New York: Harcourt, Brace.

Piaget, J. (1932). *The moral judgment of the child*. New York: Free Press.

Piaget, J. (1936). *The origins of intelligence in children*. New York: International Universities Press.

Pipp, S., Fischer, K., & Jennings, S. (1987). Acquisition of self and mother knowledge in infancy. *Developmental Psychology, 23*, 86–96.

Popper, E. (1975). The rationality of scientific revolutions. In R. Harré (Ed.), *Problems of scientific revolutions*. Oxford: Clarendon Press.

Pribram, K. (1980). Cognition and performance: The relation to neural mechanisms of consequence, confidence, and competence. In A. Routtenberg (Ed.), *Biology of reinforcement: Facets of brain stimulation reward*. New York: Academic Press.

Reiser, M. (1984). *Mind, brain, body: Toward a convergence of psychoanalysis and neurobiology*. New York: Basic Books.

Ricoeur, P. (1970). *Freud and philosophy: An essay on interpretation*. New Haven: Yale University Press.

Roazen, P. (1976). *Freud and his followers*. New York: Knopf.

Rogers, L. & Kegan, R. (1989). *Mental growth and mental health as distinct concepts in the study of developmental psychopathology: Theory, research, and clinical implications*. Presented paper.

Rossi, E. (1986). *The psychology of mind–body healing: New concepts of therapeutic hypnosis*. New York: W. W. Norton.

Ruble, D. (1983). Sex-role development. In M. H. Bornstein & M. E. Lamb (Eds.), *Developmental psychology: An advanced textbook*. Hillsdale, NJ: Erlbaum.

Samuels, A. (1985). *Jung and the post-Jungians*. London: Routledge & Kegan Paul.

Schafer, R. (1976). *A new language for psychoanalysis*. New Haven: Yale University Press.

Schafer, R. (1978). *Language and insight*. New Haven, CT: Yale University Press.

Schafer, R. (1983). *The analytic attitude*. New York: Basic Books.

Schaie, K. W. (Ed.). (1983). *Longitudinal studies of adult psychological development*. New York: Guilford Press.

Selman, R. (1980). *The growth of interpersonal understanding: Developmental and clinical analyses*. New York: Academic Press.

Sherry, J. (1989). Lingering shadows: Jungians, Freudians, and anti-Semitism. Conference held at The New School, New York, March 28, April 4, April 11, 1989. *The San Francisco Jung Institute Library Journal, 8*(4), 28–42.

Simos, B. (1979). *A time to grieve: Loss as a universal human experience.* New York: Bruner/Mazel.

Spence, D. (1982). *Narrative truth and historical truth.* New York: W. W. Norton.

Spence, D. (1987a). *The Freudian metaphor: Toward paradigm change in psychoanalysis.* New York: W. W. Norton.

Spence, D. (1987b). Turning happenings into meanings: The central role of the self. In P. Young-Eisendrath & J. Hall (Eds.), *The book of the self.* New York: New York University Press.

Sroufe, A., & Fleeson, J. (1986). Attachment and the construction of relationships. In W. Hartup & Z. Rubin (Eds.), *Relationships and development.* Hillsdale, NJ: Erlbaum.

Stern, D. (1985). *The interpersonal world of the infant.* New York: Basic Books.

Stevens, A. (1982). *Archetypes: A natural history of the self.* New York: Morrow.

Strupp, H. (1989). Psychotherapy: Can the practitioner learn from the researcher? *American Psychologist, 44*(4), 717–714.

Sullivan, H. S. (1953). *The interpersonal theory of psychiatry.* New York: W. W. Norton.

Sullivan, H. S. (1956). *Clinical studies in psychiatry.* New York: W. W. Norton.

Thurnher, M. (1983). Turning points and developmental change: Subjective and "objective" assessments. *American Journal of Orthopsychiatry, 53,* 52–60.

Tomkins, S. S. (1962). *Affect, imagery, and consciousness.* New York: Springer.

Tomkins, S. S. (1987). Shame. In D. Nathanson (Ed.), *The many faces of shame.* New York: Guilford Press.

Vaihinger, H. (1924). *The philosophy of "as if."* London: Routledge & Kegan Paul.

Vaillant, G. (1977). *Adaptation to life.* Boston: Little, Brown.

Varela, F. (1979). *Principles of biological autonomy.* New York: Elsevier-North Holland.

Vico, G. (1948). *The new science* (T. G. Bergin & M. H. Fisch, Trans.). Ithaca, NY: Cornell University Press. (Original work published 1744)

von Foerster, H. (1984). On constructing a reality. In P. Watzlawick (Ed.), *The invented reality* (pp. 41–61). New York: W. W. Norton.

Von Franz, M. (1981). *Puer aeturnus: A psychological study of the adult struggle with the paradise of childhood.* Boston, MA: Sigo Press.

Von Glasersfeld, E. (1984). An introduction to radical constructivism. In P. Watzlawick (Ed.), *The invented reality* (pp. 17–40). New York: W. W. Norton.

Vygotsky, L. (1962). *Thought and language.* Cambridge, MA: MIT Press.

Vygotsky, L. (1978). In M. Cole, S. Scribner, V. John-Steiner, & E. Souderman (Eds.), *Mind in society: The development of higher psychological processes.* Cambridge, MA: MIT Press.

Watzlawick, P. (Ed.). (1984). *The invented reality.* New York: W. W. Norton.

Weimer, W. B. (1977). A conceptual framework for cognitive psychology: Motor theories of the mind. In R. Shaw & J. Bransford (Eds.), *Perceiving, acting, and knowing* (pp. 267–311). Hillsdale, NJ: Erlbaum.

Weimer, W. B. (1982). Hayek's approach to the problems of complex phenomena: An introduction to the theoretical psychology of the sensory order. In W. B. Weimer & D. S. Palermo (Eds.), *Cognition and the symbolic processes* (Vol. 2). Hillsdale, NJ: Erlbaum.

Werner, H. (1957). The concept of development from a comparative and organismic point of view. In D. Harris (Ed.), *The concept of development*. Minneapolis: University of Minnesota Press.

Winnicott, D. W. (1958). *Collected papers*. New York: Basic Books.

Winnicott, D. W. (1965). *The maturational processes and the facilitating environment*. New York: International University Press.

Winnicott, D. W. (1971). *Playing and reality*. London: Tavistock.

Young-Eisendrath, P. (1984). *Hags and heroes: A feminist approach to Jungian psychotherapy with couples*. Toronto: Inner City.

Young-Eisendrath, P. (1985). Reconsidering Jung's psychology. *Psychotherapy, 22*(3), Fall.

Young-Eisendrath, P., & Hall, J. (1987). *The book of the self: Person, pretext, process*. New York: New York University Press.

Young-Eisendrath, P. & Wehr (1989). The fallacy of individualism and reasonable violence against women. In J. C. Brown & C. R. Bohn (Eds.), *Christianity, patriarchy, and abuse: A feminist critique*. New York: Pilgrim Press.

Young-Eisendrath, P., & Wiedemann, F. (1987). *Female authority: Empowering women through psychotherapy*. New York: Guilford Press.

Zigler, & Glick (1986). *A developmental approach to adult psychopathology*. New York: Wiley.

Index